"This is a comprehensive, clear and concise book. It is written in a manner that should put new parents at ease, by a well-known pediatrician who has cared for two generations of children."

—Lillian Beard, M.D., practicing
  pediatrician and associate clinical
  professor of Pediatrics, George
  Washington University School of
  Medicine, Washington, D.C.

Dr. Carl Robinson's
Basic Baby Care

A Guide for New Parents for the First Year

CARL D. ROBINSON, M.D., FAAP

New Harbinger Publications, Inc.

Publisher's Note

This publication is designed to provide accurate and authoritative information in regard to the subject matter covered. It is sold with the understanding that the publisher is not engaged in rendering psychological, financial, legal, or other professional services. If expert assistance or counseling is needed, the services of a competent professional should be sought.

Distributed in the U.S.A. by Publishers Group West; in Canada by Raincoast Books; in Great Britain by Airlift Book Company, Ltd.; in South Africa by Real Books, Ltd.; in Australia by Boobook; and in New Zealand by Tandem Press.

Copyright ©1998 by Carl D. Robinson, M.D., FAAP
New Harbinger Publications, Inc.
5674 Shattuck Avenue
Oakland, CA 94609

Cover design by SHELBY DESIGNS & ILLUSTRATES.
Cover photograph by Lloyd Dennis.
Edited by Tynan Northrop.
Text Design by Michele Waters.

Library of Congress Catalog Card Number: 97-75474.
ISBN 1-57224-105-5 Paperback

Printed in the United States on recycled paper.

New Harbinger Publications' Website address: www.newharbinger.com

First Printing.

To my parents, B. D. and Emily Robinson.
You have always been there for me.

Contents

Acknowledgments

In the early stages of writing this book, I learned very quickly that one needs the assistance of many other people. To all those who have generously given of their time and effort, a genuine thank you.

To my office staff—Regina Demas, R.N., PNP, Lyndrell George, and Randy Turner—I offer a particular thanks for tolerating me, especially during the editing period. They also recruited patients for the photos used in the book and contributed some of the questions, from personal experience, patients, and their colleagues.

To Robin Bourg, who first entered my manuscript into the computer—before I became reasonably computer literate.

I am especially indebted to Judy Normand, my assistant, in the rewriting and in-house editing of this book. Judy worked diligently with me in the final rewrite for publication. Much of the translation from "doctor talk" to "parent-friendly language" is a result of her efforts.

The photos were taken by both myself and Lloyd Dennis, a professional photographer. We became children again as we were literally "on the floor" with many of them and having a great time!

Thanks to Kristen Beck, acquisition editor at New Harbinger, who had the foresight to think this book was needed.

Thanks to the members of the New Harbinger staff including Kirk Johnson, Lauren Dockett, and others for their help in making this book a reality.

To my children, Carla and Michael, who taught me "close-up" pediatrics as a parent.

To the countless children and families I've had the privilege of caring for over the years.

A very special thank you goes to Tynan Northrop, my editor at New Harbinger, who kept the book on track and made it really work.

To any I've failed to mention, forgive me, and thanks.

Carl D. Robinson, M.D., FAAP

A Word from Dr. Robinson

Congratulations! You have a brand new baby—or are about to have one. NOW WHAT?? You probably could use some help with a few things, right? That's why I'm offering this book—especially for you new or about-to-be parents.

It's my job to know about babies. And because I know about babies I have come to know many fathers and fathers-to-be, and thousands of mothers and mothers-to-be, just like you. I see them every day and all of them have stories to tell and questions to ask. Some of their stories are beautiful—some tragic—but the stories are unique to the person who happens to be sitting in front of me at that particular moment.

What I've learned about parents from all of their stories is that each and every one of them is special. Each parent and their baby deserve all my attention and expertise as a doctor, which means that I need to be not *only* a doctor, but also a teacher, advisor, and most importantly, a friend.

If this is your first baby, I must tell you as your advisor that you're going to have to do a lot of growing up—FAST. Your new baby is going to need all the love, attention, and straight-thinking he or she can get in order to grow into a proud, healthy, productive member of this complicated society. Raising another human being, especially in this day, can be downright terrifying, but it's not impossible, and you can do it!

In a perfect world all babies would be blessed with a mother, a father, perhaps sisters and brothers, and a whole host of aunts, uncles, and cousins, not to mention grandparents! Unfortunately, our world is something less than perfect. This does not mean that if you *don't* have all this support you won't be able to do a great job of raising your child. All it takes is love, persistence, and a willingness to learn.

This book is meant to supplement what you already instinctively know, and add to the loving advice you've always had from your own mothers and grandmothers. It's to be used as a quick reference—with answers to some questions you may have always wanted to ask but were reluctant to do so for one reason or another. What it is *not* meant to be is a book to tell you *exactly* how to take care of your baby. You and your baby will, for the most part, find your own ways of growing and learning together.

I'm offering this information to you in a question-and-answer format, which should make it easy for you to refer to the baby-care topic you're most interested in. All of the questions included here have been asked over the years by my young patients and by their moms, their dads, their caregivers, and even their friends. Invariably, someone concerned about one of my patients will enter my office and begin a conversation with, "I know this is a stupid question, but ..." There *aren't* any stupid questions concerning the well-being of children. Stupidity enters the picture *only* if the questions are NOT asked!

What I have tried to do with this manual is to provide you and your baby with some sound, simple advice that should assist you in caring for him or her during your first year together. The only way to do that is to answer your questions as clearly and honestly as I can because, unfortunately, babies do not come with a set of instructions! And they are *very* complicated!

Babies are also miracles. They're soft and cuddly and sweet-smelling. They charm you with smiles, tug at your heart with tears, and tickle you with weird and wonderful new expressions every day. And surely no baby before or since has ever been so smart as *yours*! This is the stuff dreams are made of.

Babies are also cranky and wriggly and wet themselves regularly. They cry for no reason (as far as *you* can tell), and spit up on your best dress. Babies will sleep all day and worry you all night. They get sick and scare you to death when you can't understand what's wrong. They eat too much—or not enough. Babies sometimes don't want to be cuddled, making you think they don't even *like* you. And surely no baby has ever been so slow to do the things your friends and family say she *should* be doing by now! This is the real stuff.

If you're fortunate, the reality and the dreams will balance quite nicely; however, parents are often shocked to find themselves reeling in the *real* world of dirty diapers and colic instead of basking in the dreamland of sugar and spice and everything nice!

I believe that the dreams and reality actually do balance—most of the time—but for those crazy roller-coaster days that leave you breathless with love or panic for your child; those confused days when no book seems to have the answers you need; those days when we can only love them the best way we can ... for *those* days, we just have to take a deep breath and have confidence that with time and patience life will get back on track!

Try to remember that this first year won't be easy—nothing truly worth your time and effort is easy, but I think you'll find that the rewards for all your hard work will be immeasurable!

Ready? Relax, and let's learn more about what your baby's first year will bring.

Carl D. Robinson, M.D., FAAP

Chapter 1

Before Your Baby Is Born

Getting Ready

Before your baby is born, you will no doubt be concerned with having everything ready for her when you bring her home. And you can't *wait*! It's been nine months! You're *huge*, and clumsy, and TIRED! Except for the obvious spectacle of your misshapen body and the frantic movements inside your swollen belly, you may have started to think that this pregnancy might be just a figment of your imagination! "Won't this baby *ever* be born?" Then, some well-meaning friend or family member will innocently ask, "Are you ready?"

This question, when it pertains to childbirth, can be answered in two ways, both with complete conviction and honesty: "YES!" *and* "NO!" Yes, of *course* you're ready—physically. Mentally, you're in that gray area, somewhere between confidence that you *can* deal with this extraordinary thing that's happening to you and your body, and total panic that you may *not* be able to pull this off after all!

But take heart. You're almost there and you're in good company. Every mother I've ever met has had exactly these same feelings. Your body will soon be back to normal and you'll be wondering what on earth could have gotten you in such a panic!

One reason these feelings will fade is that you'll soon be much too BUSY to panic! Babies simply take a lot of care and make more demands on your time than you ever dreamed possible for such a little person! That's why it's so important to plan ahead as thoroughly as possible—*before* your baby is born.

Who will deliver my baby?

Your infant will be delivered by an obstetrical caregiver—a specialist in obstetrics and gynecology, general practitioner, perinatologist, or nurse midwife.

The obstetrician/gynecologist is a physician who specializes in the care of women during pregnancy and in diseases that affect the female reproductive organs. These doctors handle both routine and complicated deliveries.

The general practitioner is a family physician who is trained in a broad spectrum of medical areas including internal medicine, pediatrics, obstetrics, and surgery. These physicians can manage without complications the majority of simple pregnancies and deliveries that occur.

The perinatologist is an obstetrician who manages high-risk pregnancies. She can handle complications in both the mother and the unborn child. These doctors usually practice in large urban areas and in hospitals with sophisticated equipment.

The nurse midwife is a nurse who has specialized in obstetrics and gynecology. She is certified to care for normal, uncomplicated pregnancies and deliveries. She cannot do cesarean births or any other complicated surgical procedures.

What are the different roles of an obstetrician versus a pediatrician?

The obstetrical caregiver is responsible for the overall monitoring and care of the mother during the pregnancy and delivery. He or she is the person with whom you will discuss issues of birthing, types of delivery, and complications. She will monitor the growth of the unborn child (fetus) inside of you and give you advice on what you need to do to insure an uncomplicated delivery. Your obstetrical caregiver will be there for your delivery and will help to bring your infant into the world.

Your pediatric caregiver takes over after the infant is born. He will be responsible for the immediate care and well-being of your infant. While usually a pediatrician, he may be a family practitioner or a pediatric nurse practitioner. If any problems occur, he will be the one who will manage the problem (in the office or hospital) or he may call in another pediatric specialist.

What's the first thing I should do before the baby is born?

The first and most important thing to do is to choose a pediatrician—a doctor for your baby. Your family and friends who've used a particular doctor can be a valuable resource for referral. Your obstetrician/gynecologist, an accredited hospital, or a medical school are also excellent sources for a recommendation.

How do I know if he's a good doctor?

Ask questions! Here are some questions you should have answered—directly or indirectly:

◑ What are the doctor's medical credentials?

◑ How long has he been in practice?

◑ Does he make me feel comfortable and listen carefully to my questions?

◑ Does he *answer* my questions with respect and in a way that I can understand?

◑ Is he available (on-call) only at certain times during the day or night?

◑ Who covers for him when he's unavailable?

◑ Will the doctor or his nurse/assistant return my calls?

◑ Will I always see the doctor, or will I sometimes see his nurse or assistant?

◑ Will he respect my religious beliefs or philosophies about raising my child?

◑ How does he feel about circumcision, breast-feeding, etc.?

◑ Can he relate to me?

What if I can't afford a private doctor?

If you are not in a position to engage a private pediatrician, you may consider a clinic. Most local hospitals or social service agencies will be able to direct you to one appropriate for you and your baby. Here are a few things you may want to know before you visit the clinic:

◑   Do they accept all babies, or just children in their area, delivered by an affiliated doctor?

◑   Do they require you to make an appointment, or do they accept walk-ins?

◑   How do they want to be paid?

◑   Will you see the same doctor every time?

What are some things I need to do for myself before the baby comes?

◑   Arrange for someone to help you with the baby after you bring her home!

◑   If you work, make sure plans for maternity leave are finalized.

◑   If possible, pre-register at the hospital to save time when you arrive for admission.

◑   Make sure you have enough food in the house for a couple of weeks. It's sometimes difficult to run to the store with a newborn! It may be a good idea to find out if there are grocery stores or drug stores in your area that deliver.

What sorts of things should I take to the hospital with me?

◑   Take along a robe, slippers, two or three nightgowns, and about six pairs of underwear.

◑   All toiletries (toothbrush, makeup, etc.) you normally use at home.

◑   A favorite book (like *this* one!), magazines, address/phone book, stationery, stamps, envelopes, and your insurance card!

◑   Change for the cold drink machine, coffee (not for *you*—for your guests!), etc.

◑   A favorite (and pretty) outfit to wear home.

◑   A receiving blanket and something special for the *baby* to wear home.

◑   Take along a fairly large suitcase. You may have extra gifts to bring home!

What are some of the things I should have on hand when I bring the baby home?

In general, I suggest to parents not to overdo it. Many times, mothers will have baby showers which provide them with more than adequate clothing for the infant. Other family and friends will give personal gifts, and don't forget the still-good clothing from any older brothers and sisters or from friends' or relatives' babies!

Though the possibilities are endless, there *are* certain items I consider essential for the newborn:

- Approximately five undershirts
- Approximately three nightgowns—preferably with drawstring bottoms
- Two sleeper blankets
- Adequate diapers—newborn size! If you are using commercial diapers, have at least four dozen on hand. If you are using cloth diapers, four to six dozen should be available, with at least four pairs of waterproof pants.

If the climate and temperature warrant, you may consider:

- Two sweaters
- One hat or head covering
- A bunting (if the weather is cold)
- A snowsuit with mittens (if the weather is *very* cold!)

What are some of the toiletries I should have on hand at home?

For bathing:

- Baby soap
- "No tears" shampoo
- Baby lotion
- Three to five washcloths
- At least three terrycloth towels

I also recommend:

- Zinc oxide ointment for diaper rash
- Cotton balls

◑   Comb and brush

◑   File for baby's nails

◑   Baby nail clippers

What are the major concerns about baby furniture?

First and foremost, paint on *all* furniture should be LEAD FREE! You should also make sure that the furniture is sturdy, with no sharp edges or easily breakable parts. The furniture doesn't have to be new, just clean and in good shape!

What about using cribs and bassinets?

I do *not* recommend bassinets for children because they are too easily collapsed or tipped over. Instead, I recommend that parents use a strong, sturdy crib which can be easily cleaned. You should cover the waterproof mattress with fitted sheets and use bumper padding which can be tied securely to the crib railings. And remember: ALWAYS KEEP THE SIDES *UP* ON THE CRIB!

How do you "babyproof" a child's crib?

The baby's crib or bed should have slats that are no more than 2 3/8 inches apart. Little arms and legs may be seriously injured if caught between slats placed too far apart. The distance from the *top* of the raised railing to the *top* of the mattress should be no less than *twenty-two inches*. When the railing is lowered, the top of the railing should be at least *four inches* above the mattress.

The sheets on the mattress should be tight-fitting and there should be no toys hung over or attached to the crib that have strings or ribbons on them. The baby's natural movements could cause him to become entangled, causing serious injury or death.

It is also very important to remember that, if the baby is placed on a bed (without the protection of railings or other barriers), that you NEVER LEAVE HIM UNATTENDED! It is entirely possible for the child to somehow FALL OFF that bed!

Is there other furniture I should consider "essential"?

Other than a good, safe place for the baby to sleep, you will likely already have the things you'll need, or you will have substitutes—a countertop makes a great changing table; the kitchen or bathroom sink will make a terrific bathtub; an extra chest or cabinet painted a bright color can turn into a wonderful place for baby's clothes or toys—use your imagination! However, there is one item (not usually considered to be furniture) that, in my opinion, is essential for the safety of your child: the infant car seat.

Car Seats

Children should *never* ride in the front seat of your car, and any infant under twenty pounds or one year of age should always ride in the back seat in a rear-facing car seat. After one year of age, a front-facing car seat in the back seat is acceptable.

When should I purchase the car seat?

I believe you should have the car seat before the baby is born so that she can be assured of riding home from the hospital in safety. Though it's a nice thought to be able to hold your child in your arms on the way home, it can be *extremely* dangerous. Also, the child will be able to adjust to being in the car seat from birth, avoiding a hassle getting her into it when she's older. It will become routine for her, as using a seat belt is for you.

What should I look for when shopping for a car seat?

All car seats should meet the current Federal Motor Vehicles Safety Standards issued by the National Highway Traffic Safety Administration (NHTSA). An approved child safety seat has a label that reads: "The child restraint system conforms to all applicable Federal Motor Vehicle Safety Standards." Furthermore, the American Academy of Pediatrics will provide you with a list of car seats that meet these federal guidelines. Write AAP Publications, P.O. Box 927, Elk Grove, IL 60009-0927 (or call 1-800-443-9016).

Even with an approved car seat, it is important that you use the car seat properly to protect your baby. Here are a few things to keep in mind:

◑   Always position the baby's seat in the back seat of your vehicle.

◑   Even if the car is equipped with a passenger-side air bag, do not put an infant in the front seat. If the air-bag should suddenly inflate, the child could be seriously injured or killed. The NHTSA recommends that *all children under twelve years of age* be placed in the rear seat with restraints.

(l)   The baby's car seat should have *two* shoulder straps and a lap belt.

(l)   Make sure the car seat is secure. Belts should hold the seat firmly in place.

(l)   If a rear seat is not available in your car and an alternative is available for travel, you should use the alternative! The NHTSA states that if you have NO CHOICE, and *must* place the infant in the front seat, she should *still* be placed in a rear-facing car seat. Push the car seat as far back as possible between the child and the air bag and if you have an on-off switch, disable the air bag.

Your Baby's Doctor-To-Be: The Prenatal Visit

We encourage parents to visit their pediatrician before the delivery of the infant. This allows both the parents and doctor to get to know and understand each other, and to learn what all of you can expect from each other. Occasionally personalities do not match, or the answers to your questions will not be consistent with your own views. Since this is, in essence, an interview, you will be better able to determine whether or not this particular doctor should be entrusted with the care of your precious infant-to-be!

Also, while checking out the doctor, you'll be able to judge the quality of his office environment and his staff. Many times, the front desk space and personnel will tell volumes about the doctor's overall practice!

Allow plenty of time for this visit. You'll be meeting not only the doctor, but his nursing staff and office personnel and all of them will have questions for you!

Your partner is encouraged to accompany you to the first visit, but may be asked to join the discussion later if you have questions and concerns that you are more comfortable discussing in private with your doctor.

What kind of things will we talk about at this visit?

Some of the things you may be discussing with your doctor are:

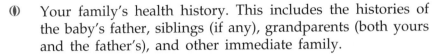

- Your family's health history. This includes the histories of the baby's father, siblings (if any), grandparents (both yours and the father's), and other immediate family.

- Is there any history of heart disease, hypertension, blood disorders (such as sickle cell anemia), or mental illness in the family?

- Have there been any problems with the pregnancy so far—emotional or physical?

- Are you taking any medication (prescription or non-prescription)?

- Any past surgeries?

- He will talk about the risk factor of sexually transmitted diseases.

- The doctor will determine, if you don't know, based on the date of your menstrual period, the baby's due date.

- Will you have a C-section or vaginal delivery?

- How do you plan to feed your baby—breast or bottle?

- Were there any previous pregnancies and what was the outcome? (Did you have a normal pregnancy and birth?)

- He'll want to know your age, marital status, and possibly your occupation. (All of this information is necessary in determining whether or not you are to be considered a high-risk patient.)

- Do you plan to raise your baby the way you were raised, or do you plan to change some things? What will you change?

- He will inquire about your health insurance and/or payment methods: Are you part of the managed health care organization he participates in? What are the limits of your coverage? The doctor should reveal, at this point, the cost of his hospital visits and approximate office visit charges. Should you need financial aid, he should be able to refer you to various sources for assistance.

- Have you been offered HIV testing?

- Do you or your partner smoke, take drugs, or drink?

- Are you concerned about being able to afford food and clothing for your baby?

◑   The doctor may ask PRIVATELY if your partner ever loses his temper or threatens you in any way. This is a concern, not only for you, but for your child.

◑   Do you plan to return to work or start a job?

That's a lot of information! What should we find out about the *doctor*?

◑   How long has the doctor been in practice?

◑   What hospital does he use?

◑   How does he handle problems that may arise during delivery, or in the nursery—and will he or an associate be available in case there are problems?

◑   How often will you bring your child in for office visits during the first year?

◑   How can you reach the doctor after hours if there is an emergency?

◑   How does he feel about circumcision?

◑   How does he feel about breast-feeding versus the bottle?

◑   Will you need vitamins or fluoride to supplement your baby's diet?

◑   What books does he recommend about caring for your child?

That seems to cover everything! Will he have some good advice for me concerning pregnancy and birth?

◑   The doctor will advise you to shop for a car seat and to use it in the back seat of the car.

◑   He will probably advise against infant walkers.

◑   A smoke-free environment is encouraged and he will advise against drinking or drugs during this time—including caffeine!

◑   It will be important for you to receive dental check-ups.

◑   Attending childbirth classes and learning infant CPR will be advised.

◑   Keeping your prenatal appointments will be strongly recommended!

- He will advise that relationships within your family will change and to prepare any other children for the birth of the new baby.

- Your doctor will tell you to anticipate some post-natal depression, fatigue, and the "baby blues."

- He will advise you to develop a support system of friends and family to help you through the first hectic weeks.

- If you need additional information or help, the doctor should be able to answer your questions or refer you to appropriate sources and/or agencies for guidance.

Chapter 2

🐎

At the Hospital

The Delivery

It's getting close to time for me to deliver. I'm scared. What should I expect to happen?

No matter how prepared you may think yourself to be for the onset of labor, you'll probably go into it without the slightest idea of its intensity! The scariest part, for most new mothers, is not being able to predict just how your body will react to labor pains; no one has ever been able to articulate just how it feels, though some graphic descriptions have been offered!

Simply put, your baby is going to be born, no matter how you feel or what you do. This loss of control, as your body and the baby take over, can be very frightening, but you must remember that it's a perfectly natural process and that it can be the most beautiful experience of your life. And any memory of *physical* pain you may have felt will disappear once you have held your baby in your arms!

Once labor begins, you must see it through! It may help if you remember that labor is really something the *baby* is going through. *You* are the instrument through which your child enters the world. Your baby, through your body's contractions and pushing, *will* make his way down the birth canal to be born!

Though this experience is new and possibly terrifying for *you*, it is much more traumatic for the *baby*, so try to keep your surroundings as calm and peaceful as possible.

In addition, it's very important that you are as prepared as you can be to help him or her into this world. Don't be afraid to ask your obstetrician for advice. She will probably tell you that a certain amount of training helps; perhaps attending birthing classes with other mothers-to-be would help you understand and cope with this new and exciting stage in your life. However, if you don't wish to attend formal childbirth classes, I would strongly recommend talking with your partner, family, obstetrician, and/or other women who've gone through the birth process. You'll find that by sharing your feelings, some of your anxiety will go away.

After the physical experience of labor, you are apt to feel very emotional and confused. For nine months you've been "about-to-be" a mother. Suddenly, after only moments, it seems, you *are*! That's a tough transition to make so quickly. You will likely be feeling extremely vulnerable, and if you have a partner, he will no doubt be going through some emotional upheavals himself because of *your* special needs. Not to mention the fact that *he's* become a father!

For nine months your body has taken care of the baby; now *you* must, and that realization can be overwhelming at first, so let your emotions flow!

You are physically and emotionally drained, your hormones are all mixed up, and you're TIRED! It's no wonder that you can't think too clearly or be overly concerned with how *other* people feel—even your new baby! But don't worry. More than likely, a few hours rest will put things back into perspective and you (and your partner or spouse) will be able to enjoy being a new parent.

What should I expect to happen in a regular delivery room?

The delivery room is a surgical suite. It is equipped for deliveries as well as emergency surgeries. For example, if the baby is lodged in the birth canal, and there is a necessity to deliver the baby by surgical means, there will be no need to change rooms. This extra measure of time saved may be critical to your infant's life. Your obstetrician may perform an episiotomy (a small cut or incision to enlarge the opening of the vagina), allowing the baby easier passage.

When the baby is ready to be born, the delivery room becomes very busy. You may have elected to have spinal or epidural anesthesia, which is done by the anesthesiologist, who is an M.D., or a nurse anesthetist, an R.N. There will be a circulating nurse in the delivery room who will provide the delivery room staff with items that may be required. Your husband, significant other, or birth partner may be in the delivery suite—in fact, I encourage this. You may also request that a mirror be placed so that you can watch the baby's actual birth!

What is a birthing room?

The concept of the delivery room has changed over the last twenty years. Now, in addition to the classic surgical suites, hospitals sometimes use birthing rooms—delivery rooms which look like regular bedrooms, but with all the necessary equipment for medical intervention. In these rooms, you and your significant other may be together during labor and delivery and enjoy the birth of your child in relative comfort.

What happens immediately after the baby is born?

One of the first things that happens is that the umbilical cord is clamped off with a wire or plastic clamp and cut. The umbilical cord is the "lifeline" attached from the baby to the placenta. The cord carries nutrients and blood from the mother to the baby before it is born.

The cord itself is shiny and white and should have three vessels, two arteries, and one vein. Some congenital anomalies (abnormal conditions that an infant is born with) may correlate, for unknown reasons, with the cord having less than two arteries and one vein. The cord is usually painted with a triple dye umbilical antiseptic which helps prevent infection and may have a blue or purplish color when you see it. The stump of the cord attached to the baby's navel will fall off within the first three weeks.

One of the most important things that occurs in the delivery room is that you'll find out just how much your baby weighs. In my experience, questions related to the weight of the baby (second only to whether it's a boy or girl!) is uppermost in the minds of parents. Footprints and fingerprints are also taken at this time, and ID bands are placed on the baby's wrist and ankle.

Why is the ID band so important?

Shortly after your baby is stabilized by the nurses in the delivery suite, one of them will place this band on your child. In doing so, she will check *your* name band to make sure it's the same as the baby's. This banding is very important, as it identifies the child as *yours*. You wouldn't want to go home with the wrong baby!

What are some of the things the doctor will look for to make sure my baby is okay?

The first thing the delivery staff will concern itself with are the "ABCs": "A" stands for airway—seeing that your child has an open airway for breathing. The infant will be suctioned to remove all the mucus and fluid received as a result of the delivery process. "B" stands for breathing. Once the airway is open, we look and listen to the breath sounds. "C" represents cardiac or heart, which is checked for rate and rhythm.

Then an APGAR assessment is done. The APGAR scoring method was created in 1953 by Dr. Virginia Apgar, an anesthesiologist, who measured babies' circulatory activity, respiratory activity, muscle tone, and reflex and assigned each a number on a scale of 0 to 10. Dr. Apgar found a correlation between the medical condition of the infant and the total number scored on the APGAR scale. The letters APGAR, in addition to being the name of the doctor who invented the method, stand for: Appearance, Pulse, Grimace, Activity, and Respiration (see chart on page 21).

Appearance refers to the coloring of the child: we check the color of the skin, lips, and the mucous membranes on the inside of the mouth for abnormal coloring. Pulse refers to the heartbeat, which should be strong and steady. Grimace refers to the reflex movements of the child. Activity is the measure of the muscle tone of the infant, and Respiration measures breathing.

APGARs are measured during the *first* minute of life, and in the *fifth* minute after the child is born. Take, for example, a newborn with the following scores: appearance (pale) = 1; pulse rate present but less than 100 = 1; no grimace (facial expression) = 0; some movement of the lower extremities = 1; respiratory rate is 20 = 1. The total APGAR score for this baby is 4, indicating some potential problems. The child is stimulated, given oxygen, and warmed up before the five minute APGAR is done. Hopefully, this APGAR score will be improved. Remember, the lower the number of the APGAR score, the more serious the condition of the child.

We usually consider scores of 7–10 (10 being the highest score) as reflecting relatively good condition; 4–6 is in fair condition; and, from 0–4, poor condition requiring immediate attention. The APGAR score is believed more important at five minutes than at one minute. At one minute, the APGAR indicates whether intervention needs to take place immediately; the five minute score reinforces those findings and helps influence what type of care is needed. The chart below should give you some idea of what the APGAR scores mean:

APGAR Scores—How Doctors Measure Your Baby's Health Status at Birth

Sign	0	1	2
Appearance	Pale or blue	Pink body, blue extremities	Pink extremities
Pulse	Can't detect	Rate less than 100	Above 100
Grimace	Doesn't respond	Grimace	Good cry to stimuli
Activity	Weak or flaccid	Some movement	Good movement of extremities
Respiration	Not breathing	Slow breathing	Good or irregular breaths

While APGAR scores are good tools for quick assessment, the most important tool is close monitoring and reevaluation of the baby by the hospital staff in the first hours of life!

After the APGAR assessment, the nurse attending the baby will place it in an incubator or under an overhead warmer in order to maintain the temperature in a normal range. If problems are present or anticipated, the pediatrician or neonatologist (a pediatric newborn specialist) may be called in or may already be present.

My baby swallowed some dark stuff during delivery and had some breathing problems. What happened?

Your baby swallowed some *meconium*, the greenish-black, tarlike stuff that was in the baby's intestinal tract. A small percentage of infants will have a bowel movement before birth (approximately 10 percent). Of that group, those who pass a small amount usually don't have any problems. The infants who pass a large amount of meconium and swallow it may have some respiratory problems. This is called meconium aspiration. In the delivery room, your doctor is very alert for the presence of meconium and, if present, will suction (a gentle withdrawing of fluid via an aspirator or through a tube which is connected to a syringe or to a vacuum machine) your infant at birth. If this doesn't help, these babies are turned over to the pediatrician or neonatologist for further care as they may become very ill.

Why is the baby given Vitamin K?

All newborns are born with a low level of Vitamin K, which is necessary for blood clotting. Vitamin K is given to avoid bleeding problems that can occur with your baby shortly after birth. Bleeding as a result of Vitamin K deficiency is rare, occurring in only 1 in 4,000 infants.

I've heard people say that the blood from the umbilical cord is studied. Why?

If there is a family history of some genetic, metabolic, or blood problem, some blood from the cord is taken and studied. Additionally, some babies are born with excessive blood loss and some mothers are profoundly anemic (have low blood counts). This needs to be known so that corrective measures can be instituted.

What other sorts of screening tests are done?

There are some screening studies mandated by law and are done in order to protect your child. These studies may include a thyroid examination, a bilirubin (a chemical in the blood that results from used-up red blood cells) test, a blood typing, or a complete blood count (CBC). In addition, the following tests are commonly done in the United States:

Sickle-cell Anemia: This disorder is part of a group of genetic (inherited) blood disorders that occur primarily in those of African American descent. "Sickle-cell" refers to the crescent shape that some red blood cells become, which inhibits the carrying of oxygen in the blood properly. While the occurrence of sickle cell is found in 8–10 percent of the African American population, sickle-cell anemia occurs only when a large proportion or majority of red blood cells sickle, in approximately 1 in 400 African Americans. Children with sickle-cell anemia may, after six to nine months of life, be seen with swelling of the extremities, pain, and a low blood count.

Phenylketonuria (PKU): This condition is screened usually after the first twenty-four hours of life. It is repeated by your pediatrician at your first office visit. The latest the repeat study should be done is the third week of life. In the overall population, PKU occurs in 1:12000 infants.

PKU is a genetic problem which is caused by a lack of a liver enzyme called hepatic phenylalanine hydroxylase. This can result in mental retardation and seizures in most affected children. When caught early, this problem can be treated effectively with a special diet.

Hypothyroidism: The primary result of hypothyroidism (a lowered [hypo] thyroid level) is mental retardation and a delayed-to-poor growth. If discovered early, this can be treated with oral medication and the children will lead reasonably normal lives. Hypothyroidism occurs in 1 out of every 4000 infants.

Galactosemia: This is another genetic disorder, rare in African Americans, that occurs when there is an absence of a liver enzyme. These infants may be normal at birth and subsequently develop vomiting, diarrhea, and failure to thrive. Although this disease is rare, occurring in only 1 in 62,000 births, if not discovered early, infants usually die within the first six weeks of either liver failure or bacterial infection in the bloodstream. The treatment is the elimination of dietary galactose by withholding foodstuff with galactose present. An example would be to give soy formula with sucrose to replace lactose (milk) in the formula.

Hearing: Hearing is also screened in many states, on all infants. This is strongly endorsed, as the earlier your doctor is able to identify hearing problems, the better the outcome. The test is quick, painless, and relatively inexpensive.

What are some of the major things the doctor is looking for when he checks the baby in the hospital?

The pediatrician does a thorough examination in the nursery. He makes sure the weight is fine and listens to the lungs and heart for abnormalities. He checks the baby's eyes for cataracts, looks at the genitalia for deformity, feels the stomach for any enlarged organs, and checks the hips and extremities for dislocation and deformity.

Why are drops or ointment put in my baby's eyes?

You and your pediatrician can agree to delay the drops/ointment for a few minutes if you wish to establish good eye-to-eye contact with your baby right after birth. However, it will be necessary for the delivery room nurse specialist who cares for your child to put an antibiotic ointment or solution in the baby's eyes. This is done to avoid some types of infectious diseases that may be passed to the baby's eyes during delivery.

The doctor said the baby has an umbilical hernia. What is this?

Umbilical hernias (a protrusion around the navel) are a result of a weakness of the muscles in the anterior abdominal wall and are not uncommon. They occur most frequently among African American infants for unknown reasons. What I emphasize to parents is that the vast majority of these hernias are minor and will "go away" by the time the child is three years old. The hernias that do not resolve themselves are usually surgically removed at the appropriate time, most often for cosmetic reasons. African American mothers have a long history of using bellybands with fifty-cent pieces taped over the baby's navel! Please don't do this! There is a high risk of both infection and severe skin irritation with these practices. Just leave it alone and it will go away!

People talk a lot about what color the baby's eyes will be and whether or not he or she will have "good" or "bad" hair. What can I expect?

First of all, the way your baby looks depends entirely on genetics! Most African American infants, for example, have either brown, light brown, or hazel (greenish) eyes. Rarely will there be other colors, but it *does* happen. It depends upon the baby's mother and father, *and* upon whether or not there is some past connection with a person of another race. In this case, you may well see an African American infant with blue eyes! Again, this is genetics at work. Baby's eyes, however, will not assume a permanent color until later in the first year of life.

As for the baby's hair ... I believe we need to get away from terms such as "good" and "bad" when referring to hair. Hair texture, like the eye color, is usually a result of one's heredity. Mothers and fathers with straighter hair will generally have children with the same type of hair; the same for kinky or curled hair. Coarse hair or curly hair in parents will usually result in the same for the child.

As with the texture of hair, many infants will have varying amounts of hair on the head—from very little, to a great deal. It should not be cause for concern, as most of the hair that the baby is born with will fall out during the first year of life. The texture of the hair also changes with the permanent replacement hair.

During Your Hospital Stay

I've heard a lot about "rooming-in" while in the hospital. What is this?

Many mothers, especially the ones who choose to breast-feed, have the babies "room in" with them; i.e., the babies are in the mother's room twenty-four hours a day. This allows the mother (you) to be immediately responsive to your baby's needs. If your hospital does not allow this procedure, make sure the staff knows that your child is to be brought to you when she is hungry. Some moms ask for an early discharge, if the rooming-in service is not available, so that they can be more in control of the situation.

I hear a lot about "bonding" with my baby. What if it doesn't happen for me?

"Bonding" is just another catchword meaning to seal or *bond* a relationship; get the *feel* of it; forge a loving, lifelong connection with someone. The problem stems from the fact that much of the literature concerning "bonding" tends to give you the impression that it should happen *instantly*, and if it doesn't, then you're possibly lacking some very basic and essential human feelings!

In my opinion, this assessment is premature and not necessarily true. The feelings *are* there—just new and undeveloped. Physically, the both of you have been "attached" to each other and felt each other's presence for nine months—*mentally*, you've just met!

So you're *not* experiencing the ecstatic, "I've never felt this kind of love before" emotion you've read and heard about. Why should you?

Simply put, your baby is exactly what he or she appears to be: a baby. The infant has not yet become a *person*, a human being who recognizes you as his mother! As a newborn, he reacts only to his immediate needs—food, warmth, and TLC. His distinct personality, the thing that will bring all those special "bonding" feelings to the surface, will develop as he ages and as the two of you get to know each other.

However, I'd like to add that the most sensitive time for the *physical* aspect of bonding is immediately after birth. Have the doctor or nurse bring your child to you so that you may touch her and make eye contact. This period immediately after birth appears to be a highly receptive time for both mother and child. The touching and stroking and the sound of both your voices will be comforting to you and your child. However, if you are too exhausted after labor—don't worry. Just take your baby in your arms as soon as you feel up to it. The process of bonding will happen naturally and the love and connection between the two of you will *not* be lost!

How long should I stay in the hospital?

Until recent years, the standard length of stay was three days for a regular delivery, and five days for a C-section. This time has been reduced significantly with the advent of new health systems and emphasis on cost savings. Furthermore, these time periods were probably not based on strong scientific principles. The current standard is approximately forty-eight hours for a regular delivery, three to four days for a C-section. This allows time for the baby to settle in and stabilize, giving the doctors the opportunity to make sure everything is all right. It also allows your doctor to see that you have developed no complications and are ready for discharge home with your new baby.

What are some of the problems that my baby may have that would keep him in the hospital longer than usual?

Some of the other problems may include: meconium aspiration, transient respiratory distress, jaundice, infections, and feeding difficulty.

What is the purpose of the birth certificate?

Every birth in the United States is supposed to be recorded and documented. Birth certificates vary from state to state; however, certain recorded information is universal: the names and ages of the baby's parents, date of birth and citizenship, selected questions about the pregnancy, place of birth, sex, race, and name of the child. Other information may be required by the baby's state of birth. This is an important document, as it validates your infant's birth—make sure the information is correct! Check especially the spelling of your child's name.

Although this important information is kept on file in the Vital Records department of the state health department, please keep an official copy of the birth certificate in a safe place for your family!

Circumcision

Circumcision is both controversial and emotional and has been since its beginning over 3,500 years ago! The American Academy of Pediatrics Task Force on Circumcision stated in 1989 that "newborn circumcision has potential medical benefits and advantages as well as disadvantages and risks. When circumcision is being considered, the benefits and risks should be explained to parents and informed consent obtained."

If you decide to have a circumcision done, then I recommend the following:

◑   Wait until after the first day of birth—give the baby's body some time to stabilize.

◑   Make sure your pediatrician has examined the baby and is assured he is healthy and ready for circumcision.

◑   Don't circumcise until the baby has urinated at least once!

Circumcision does prevent problems that may result from the inability to pull the foreskin back. It also prevents inflammation of the head (glans) of the penis as well as the opening of the penis. The reduction in the number of urinary tract infections is inconclusive, though it would appear that removal of the foreskin eliminates an ideal place for bacteria to thrive.

Also in the United States, circumcision appears to all but eliminate the possibility of cancer of the penis. It does not appear to make any difference in reducing sexually transmitted diseases.

I must tell you, however, that there are pediatricians who believe that circumcision is both unnatural and unnecessary. These pediatricians feel that with the teaching and exercise of proper hygiene and care, the risks of infection and penile cancer would be minimal. Whether your child should or should not have a circumcision is an entirely personal matter which should be based on your basic beliefs, religious or otherwise, and a comprehensive discussion of the pros and cons of circumcision with your doctor before and after your male infant is born.

Multiple Births

And then there were two . . . or three, or four—or more! With the new fertility drugs on the market, seemingly any number is possible. However, we will limit our discussion to twins.

What is meant by "fraternal" or "identical" twins?

Twins are either monozygotic (conceived by one egg) or dizygotic (conceived by two eggs). Monozygotic twins are called "identical"; dizygotic twins are "fraternal."

If the babies are of different sex, then they are not, obviously, identical and are called fraternal or same-date babies. However, doctors sometimes have difficulty, in the delivery room, determining whether or not babies are identical if they are of the same sex. The diagnosis of whether the babies are identical or fraternal is made by the examination of the placenta.

How often do twins occur?

Twins constitute a small percentage of all births but account for a significant percentage of all prenatal deaths. Therefore, a woman expecting twins (identical or fraternal) should be followed closely by her obstetrician.

Your Newborn's Five Senses

Though your new baby's senses are not as sharp as they will soon become, they are probably much more sensitive than you imagine!

Sight: Though the baby's vision is not perfect at birth, he can see, and his vision will improve dramatically at about one month of age and continue to progress from there. Just make sure to make eye contact with him as often as possible. You may also attach an unbreakable mirror in the crib, along with bright-colored or black and white shapes to stimulate vision.

Hearing: Naturally, your baby, if normal, can hear when she's born and her hearing will become more sensitive as she ages. Mom's heartbeat will comfort her and she will definitely respond to loud or irritating noises! Parents should not use "baby talk," but only *slow* their speech slightly.

Smell: The baby's sense of smell is very well developed at birth. He will be able to recognize mom's "smell" within the first forty-eight hours!

Taste: The newborn's taste buds are naturally "milk oriented" and he will be able to distinguish mom's breast milk from other milk! He will also let you know, with a grimace, when tasting something he doesn't like!

Touch: The baby will almost immediately be able to recognize the touch of different people. He should also be stroked and massaged gently with the fingertips. However, I do suggest that parents not overdo the touching, as the newborn's skin is very sensitive.

Your Newborn's Reflexes

I understand the doctor will check my baby's reflexes. What are the different types?

Your pediatrician will do a neurological examination noting the various reflexes—ones all babies are born with. The basic reflexes are:

Rooting Reflex: This reflex has evolved from the primitive human and enables the baby to find the nipple at feeding time. At birth, the baby will "root" from side to side. After about four months this reflex will disappear and she'll simply turn her head and move her mouth into a position to be able to suck.

Grasp Reflex: This is another primitive survival reflex. It may be seen even before birth through the ultrasound procedure, and babies are often seen sucking on their thumbs or toes! After birth, this reflex may be elicited by placing a finger or nipple in the baby's mouth and touching the roof of the mouth. The baby will automatically begin to suck. This reflex allows the baby to place his mouth around the areola of the nipple and squeeze the nipple between his tongue and palate, causing the milk to be forced out. The tongue actually moves from the areola to the nipple, creating a negative pressure, which secures the nipple in the baby's mouth. This reflex will disappear after the first year.

Moro Reflex: This happens when the baby's head changes positions or falls backward, or if the baby is startled: he will throw his arms and legs out and extend his neck, bringing his arms together and crying very loudly! This reflex will last for about two months.

Tonic Neck Reflex: This reflex resembles a fencing posture. If the baby's head is turned to one side, the arm on that side of his body will straighten and the opposite arm will bend, as if fencing. It will disappear after about seven months.

Plantar Reflex: Stroke the sole of the baby's foot; toes will curl and the foot will flex. This reflex will disappear after about one year.

Palmar Reflex: Stroke the palm of the hand; she will immediately grasp your finger (for about the first year).

Walking or Stepping Reflex: If you hold the baby under the arms and let the soles of his feet touch a flat surface, he will touch one foot in front of the other, giving the appearance of walking. This reflex will disappear after about two months.

Chapter 3

At Home

The Basics

Now that you have your baby home and everything is in order (sort of!), we need to tackle the practical, hands-on aspect of baby care—picking up, putting down, and everything in between, which, as you will see, can be a bit mind-boggling! With a little advance planning and a lot of patience, however, you'll amaze yourself at how quickly you'll become proficient in the fine art of "baby rearing"!

Picking Up and Holding Your Baby

What's the best way to pick up and hold my baby?

It's amazing how complicated such a simple act as picking up your baby can seem at first! A tiny, sometimes squirmy baby can become a major test of your physical and mental abilities! Just remember to relax and go slowly. Your baby will be only as calm as *you* are!

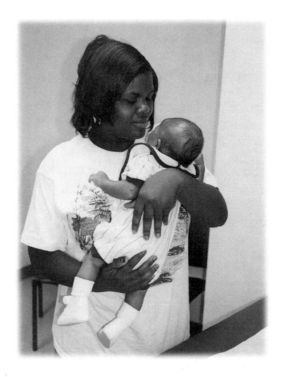

The first and most important rule is: ALWAYS MAKE SURE THE BABY'S HEAD IS SUPPORTED FIRST, THEN THE REST OF THE BODY.

A WORD OF CAUTION:

After you've become comfortable in picking up and holding your child, sometimes there is a tendency to become careless as you pick them up! Don't forget to always pick up your baby slowly and with care, never jerking or shaking! The baby can be injured permanently by shaking or jerking the head back and forth. The delicate blood vessels inside the head can be broken, causing irreversible nerve damage.

Occasionally, you will feel very frustrated by your baby. This is perfectly normal; however, if you find that this anger or frustration appears to be increasing, find some one to look after the baby for a short period until you have calmed down. Remember, your baby has no defense against your emotions or actions. You must NEVER VENT FRUSTRATION OR ANGER BY SHAKING OR JERKING THE BABY!

List of Things to Do

It often seems that, no matter what we do, something is always forgotten, or there's something we intended to do but didn't. This is perfectly understandable; you've had a lot on your mind! Here are a couple of things to consider after you're home and more or less settled down:

- If you have not already done so, try to arrange for someone to help you with the baby for a couple of days (or more!).

- Schedule your child's first appointment with the pediatrician—usually at about two to three weeks of age. Ask for a height and weight chart to keep track of your baby's progress along with the doctor.

- If finances allow, now's the time to send out those birth announcements!

- Keep a baby book—a notebook where you can record your baby's important milestones—and fill it out as completely as possible. If you do not have a regular "baby book," use a school notebook, but write it down! Later on, you'll be glad you did!

- Create a list of important phone numbers, numbers of people you may need to call and in whom you have complete confidence. (Doctor, parents, baby-sitter, etc.)

Bathing and Diapers

Many patterns of behavior you develop in caring for your baby during the first months will continue to serve you well all through the first year. Learning the basics of such things as bathing and diapering will give you a good foundation to build on as you learn new things.

Should the baby have a bath every day?

While everyone appreciates a squeaky-clean baby, the child does not have to be bathed on a daily basis during the first several months of life. It is important, however, to do what is called "spot cleaning" or "sponge baths" on a daily basis. This will usually be necessary only after feedings and/or diaper changes. There should be NO full tub baths until the umbilical cord has fallen off and the navel has healed completely. Furthermore, if your baby is a male, and has had a circumcision, it too must be completely healed. A bath is recommended every two to three days (personally, I recommend every two days) for babies who are not yet crawling, or who are not in very dirty environments.

Do you have some general instructions for bathing?

The first rule is to make sure *you* have enough time to be able to take your time when bathing your child. The second is: BE PREPARED! Make sure everything is set up beforehand in the bathing area (the kitchen or bathroom sink make excellent "tubs" for little bodies) to eliminate excessive movements, thereby protecting your child.

Bathing is most often a pleasurable time for babies. Nice, lukewarm water in a warm room (preferably with a room temperature of 75–80 degrees for a naked baby) and your soft touch will probably be soothing to him. However, some babies will be absolute terrors to handle at bath time! But whether the first baths go smoothly, or turn into battles, it's important that you get this done, as a clean baby has a better chance of staying free of many illnesses.

What do I need to bathe my baby?

Prepare the necessary "equipment" even before undressing your baby:

◑   One or two washcloths
◑   Towels—one to lay him on; one to dry
◑   Soap—should be mild and fragrance free
◑   Shampoo—should be mild and "no tears"
◑   Warm water—do the elbow or wrist test. The water should feel WARM, not hot, to your elbow or wrist (about 75–80 degrees).

How do I give a sponge bath?

In spite of the name, most sponge baths don't use sponges, but cotton balls, small towels, or wipes. The sponge bath allows us to clean all of the important parts of the new baby without doing a full-fledged tub bath, which babies really don't need until later. A sponge bath allows you to focus on the areas that are dirty—usually the eyes, nose, ears, and bottom. Those areas should be gently wiped and dried and do not require lotion or oil after cleaning. Since you do not have to set up a tub or all of the materials associated with a full bath, a sponge bath is a quick and easy way to keep baby clean. Remember:

◑ Wash clean areas on your baby first, then the dirty areas

◑ Use only a little soap unless your baby sweats a lot

◑ Be careful not to get the umbilical stump or exposed, circumcised penis wet

What about washing his head—and the "soft spots"?

With most babies, I recommend washing the scalp using "no tears" shampoo. I do not recommend that you use oils or lotions on the baby's head unless it is extremely dry, then only sparingly.

Using the "no tears" shampoo and a wash cloth, gently wash the scalp and rinse with warm water. Don't worry about the "soft spots"! Gentle washing will not hurt your baby's head. Make sure you get all the soap rinsed off and then dry thoroughly.

What's the best way to give a full bath?

Prepare the "tub" with no more than two inches of luke-warm water (elbow or wrist test), and gather the supplies listed above.

Undress your baby gently and slowly. After lowering him into the tub of water, support his neck and head with one hand and wash him gently with the other. Remember to wash from clean areas of his body to the dirty areas—and HOLD ON! Wet, soapy babies are very slippery. After the bath, dry and wrap the baby with a soft, clean towel, then dress appropriately.

Is it good to use lotion or powder?

Your baby has a good "baby smell" already; it's really not necessary to use powders or lotions to make them smell good! If you must do this, use a SMALL AMOUNT, as some babies have very sensitive skin and even the mildest soaps and lotions may irritate. Also, there is a possibility that the child may inhale powder, creating some breathing problems. Also, I have noted some African American moms heavily oiling their baby's skin, creating a myriad of rashes! Again, USE SPARINGLY!

What about "baby wipes"?

I prefer using warm towels. Commercial baby wipes may irritate your baby's sensitive skin—and they're COLD!

How do I clean my baby's ears?

Most pediatricians will tell you that to use *anything* but a washcloth to clean the baby's ears is dangerous. In my practice I have had to remove Q-Tip ends and cotton balls from small ears and have seen cuts and scratches inside the ears caused by hairpins. In addition, wax often has to be removed because the use of Q-Tips and hairpins has pushed the wax farther back into the ear canal, causing problems for the child.

My advice is to wash (with a washcloth) only the part of the ear that you can see! If you think your child has too much wax in his ear, have your doctor take a look.

How should I clean my child's nose?

Your baby's nose does not require any special cleaning. Just wipe any drainage with a soft hand towel. As with the ears, I do not recommend putting anything inside the nose, such as swabs, fingernails, or any other handy item! There are many blood vessels inside the nose and a very thin membrane covering those vessels. Any poking or prodding may cause damage to the baby's nose or those blood vessels.

How should I clip the baby's nails?

Most babies have long fingernails at birth and they continue to grow very quickly, oftentimes resulting in scratches on your baby's face.

Personally, I believe nail clipping should be done by two people—one to secure the baby in a comfortable position, and one to actually clip the nails without having to also hold the baby.

Clippers should have rounded edges which are made especially for babies. You may also want to have an emery board for filing any sharp edges. When you clip the nails, make sure that you push the pad of the finger down a little in order to avoid cutting the finger. File any sharp edges that are too close to clip.

Please give me some basics on diaper changing!

◑ Have an area in your home which may be used as a changing area. This could be in the bathroom, or in the kitchen on an empty countertop; pad the countertop with a thick towel or foam padding that can be removed and washed.

- ⦿ First of all, obviously, you should have a clean, dry diaper—cloth or disposable, whichever you've decided to use.

- ⦿ Have a couple of small towels or washcloth handy for washing and drying. Also, you may need some cotton balls and alcohol, especially if the baby is under one month of age, to be able to wipe around the umbilical stump.

- ⦿ *Make sure your hands have been washed clean,* and if you're using cloth diapers, be very careful with the pins!

- ⦿ If the baby has had a bowel movement, it should be wiped with the soiled diaper first. This diaper should then be folded and put into a plastic bag or container for disposal or washing. (If the diaper is cloth, you may have to rinse it in the toilet before putting it into the plastic bag.) Get a clean soft hand towel and slightly moisten it and wipe the baby's genital/rectal area carefully.

- ⦿ If your baby is a girl, make sure you wipe her vaginal/rectal area from *front to back* to avoid getting particles from the rectum into the vagina.

- ⦿ Use warm water on your towel, and make sure the creases around the legs and bottom are wiped clean and dried thoroughly.

- ⦿ After the baby is clean, diaper her slowly, with care.

- ⦿ If the baby's umbilical stump is present, make sure the diaper does not cover the stump. Fold the diaper down, away from the stump. Wipe the stump of the cord with a cotton ball soaked in alcohol.

- ⦿ We have found it useful to advise parents to make sure a little boy's penis is facing downward, so that when he wets, the urine will seep downward into the diaper and not up, wetting other clothing! Also, if your son has been circumcised, wash the penis gently with soap and warm water.

What are some of the things I should consider when deciding which kind of diaper to use?

Parents often ask me if they should use cloth or disposable diapers. There are advantages and disadvantages to both. This is getting to be a question asked less and less each day. The majority of parents in the United States use disposable diapers on their infants.

If you use cloth diapers and launder them yourself, obviously, the cost will be less and you can use the diapers for a longer period of time, especially if you purchase square diapers that can be folded to fit your child as she grows larger. However, the use of cloth diapers may present some difficulties in traveling or if your child will be sent to a day care center.

While disposable diapers offer convenience for packing and traveling, they *do* cost about twice the amount of cloth diapers. These disposable diapers also keep the moisture in well, and you may have to change them more frequently than cloth, which may keep you busy going back and forth to the store just to keep the supply at a reasonable level! **(You'll need between 70–100 disposable diapers every week; 36–60 cloth diapers per week.)** Also, though they are termed "disposable," they are actually quite difficult to dispose of, environmentally; they are slow to decompose and last for years! Additionally, it is illegal to dispose of human waste; therefore, you may be required to rinse the diapers in the toilet, just as with cloth diapers.

The best feature of the disposable diaper can also be its worst feature: due to the absorbent gel found in disposables, your baby may feel dry when touched, giving you the idea that the baby is not urinating often enough. Furthermore, because you have to frequently check the diaper area, there is also a risk of introducing germs from your finger to the genital area of the baby or even transmitting germs from the baby's skin to you.

All things considered, the conveniences of disposables seem to outweigh those of cloth diapers, although ultimately the cloth versus disposable question is up to you.

What about plastic pants?

These "rubber" pants, used to control leaking, usually have elastic around the waist and legs. As a result, there is very little air circulation, which can contribute to the occurrence of frequent diaper rashes. However, if you are using cloth diapers, the plastic pants can be quite helpful and necessary in keeping the baby from soiling his clothes, especially when traveling away from home.

How do diaper services work?

If you decide to use cloth diapers and can afford it, a diaper service is excellent. The service will provide the diapers, according to the baby's size and weight; they'll pick up the soiled diapers, prepare and clean the diapers with special soaps, and return the clean and folded diapers right to your door! Also, the cost remains the same, regardless of the size of the infant. However, there are relatively few of these services available.

What's the best way to clean cloth diapers?

◗ THE MOST IMPORTANT THING IS TO WASH THE DIAPERS IN THE HOTTEST WATER POSSIBLE!

◗ Rinse the diapers in the toilet, if necessary, and wring out before putting them into a diaper pail with a fitted top.

◗ If possible, SOAK the diapers for four to six hours before washing.

◗ Depending on the number of diapers in the pail, fill about one half full of water, adding about one half cup of bleach. You may need to use less water; just make sure all the diapers are covered to soak properly.

◗ Remove the diapers from the pail after soaking and drain excess liquid before putting them into the washing machine. If you don't have space to drain, you may toss the diapers into the washer on the "spin" cycle to remove the soaking solution.

◗ If you have not soaked the diapers, add them to your next wash; i.e., WASH AS SOON AS POSSIBLE!

◗ If your baby has sensitive skin, rinse the diapers twice.

◗ I recommend you wash the diapers with a mild soap instead of a detergent. This will leave the diapers and all the baby's clothes feeling much softer.

◗ The standard drying method is tumbling in the automatic dryer, although drying outside on the line is fine, too. I don't recommend using fabric softener (sheets or liquids), as some chemicals in these products have been known to irritate the baby's skin.

How often should I change the baby's diapers?

Try to be prompt in changing your child's diapers. Of course, this will depend upon the child, but the importance of regular diaper changes cannot be stressed enough! If a baby stays wet for any period of time, not only will the wetness soak his other clothes, he will be extremely uncomfortable and proceed to let everyone know it!

Also, I suggest very strongly that you accumulate dirty, disposable diapers in a plastic bag to be disposed of later in the day. Cloth diapers should be placed in a pail (bucket) that can be cleaned later in the day, or they may also be placed in a plastic bag for later washing.

If you are away from home, it's always a good idea to have an extra set of clothes for your child, as the ones he's wearing can be soiled very quickly and easily.

Sleeping

It is important to remember that your child will sleep when *she* needs to and not just because you think she *ought* to! Her schedule will happen naturally, not because of something you do or do not do. Her body will adjust to what *her* needs are, not yours, initially; however, over time you and she will make mutual adjustments that will work. Meanwhile, let her be awake to enjoy being near you—to just *watch* you during your day. Grab a nap when she does—the housework can wait! The baby will be more peaceful and rested and so will you! It is just as important that you get adequate sleep. Remember, lack of sleep affects your brain activity: your ability to concentrate, reason, and make decisions are all affected—even your speech may be impaired! When you notice this, seek help, rest, and sleep.

When and how much will my baby sleep?

Your baby will most likely sleep quite a lot in the first few weeks of life; sometimes as much as sixteen to twenty hours per day. Take advantage of this extended sleeping time as much as you can—try to catch up on *your* sleep by napping when she does. Unfortunately, the new infants don't follow a strict pattern. They don't sleep all night. They will wake to eat, then drift back to sleep when they are full. Many babies will even drop off to sleep while they're eating. You may have to gently wake them to finish the feeding. By the time they're three or four weeks old, babies will usually begin to stay awake for longer periods of time (sleeping about fifteen to sixteen hours daily).

The waking and sleeping times will vary depending upon the infant and its age. Some babies will be alert two or three hours a day and sleep most of the rest; some will awake in the morning and sleep in the afternoon; and others will sleep for four or five hours, then be awake for one or two hours at a time. But BE PATIENT! Your baby will work out his own schedule and, eventually, it will be more or less the same as your own. Around four months, most babies will have adapted a more reasonable sleep pattern, sleeping more at night and waking during the day.

Average Sleep for Babies Based on Age

Age	Hours of sleep per 24 hours
Newborn	18
3 months	15
9 months	14
1 year	14

When should the baby have his own room or sleeping area?

If your baby is not already in her own room by the time she's three to five months old, I recommend moving her then, if at all possible. Babies, as a rule, are light sleepers. If she's in the room with you, every move *you* make, every rustle of the sheets, will wake her!

Furthermore, it has been my experience that most babies moved out of the parents' room at an early age grow accustomed to not having parents around when it's time to sleep. Also, when the parents have to go out, separation is easier for both parents and child!

Are night-lights all right?

Night-lights are fine—do whatever is comfortable for your baby; but for the most part, sleeping is just an adaptation process that your baby will work through.

What if the baby cries every time I put her down?

If your child cries a lot when put down for bed, certainly you should make sure she feels that there is nothing to be afraid of and that you are there if she needs you. You may try sitting at the bedside with the baby until she falls asleep; maybe sing a song, rub her back, or just talk gently to her. She's in her own room now and that's a big step forward—for EVERYONE!

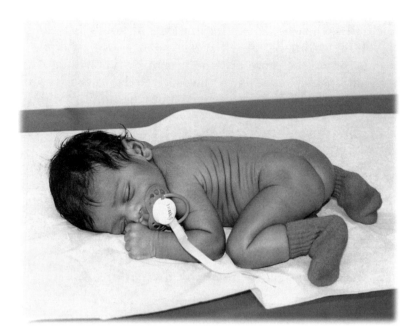

Should my baby sleep on his stomach?

There has been significant controversy in the pediatric community as to the best position for the baby to sleep. Current recommendations are that infants should be placed on their sides or back for sleep. Preliminary information shows a reduction in the SIDS events in these children.

What is SIDS?

An expert committee of the National Institute of Health in 1986 formally defined SIDS as "the sudden death of an infant under one year of age which remains unexplained after a thorough investigation, including a performance of complete autopsy, examination of the death scene and review of the clinical history." Thousands of papers have been written on SIDS and hundreds of theories on the cause have been postulated. SIDS is a worldwide problem with an incidence between 1/1000 live births. The incidence, of course, depends on how SIDS is defined in a particular country. What we do know about SIDS is that males have a higher incidence than females, with most deaths occurring between the first and fifth months, with a peak incidence at about three months of age. SIDS occurs most commonly during the winter months.

Some Risk Factors for SIDS

Maternal

◑   Young mothers < twenty years of age

◑   Anemia

◑   Poor prenatal care

◑   Poor living situation

◑   Low educational level

◑   Cigarette smoking during pregnancy

Newborn Risk Factors

◑   African American, Native American

◑   Male

◑   Premature

◑   Small for gestational age

One theory about the cause of SIDS is that these belly-sleepers may vomit, then inhale the vomit while sleeping on their stomachs. Other researchers have found an increase in carbon monoxide poisoning caused by the child inhaling the carbon dioxide breathed *out* and which has settled in the ruffled sheets and pillows. There are numerous other findings in babies that sleep on their stomachs. Even though the information is not as strong as many pediatricians would like, we are strongly recommending that babies do *not* sleep on their stomachs, but on their backs or sides. Current statistics are showing some reduction in the number of cases of SIDS with this new policy in place. We also recognize that this is not the complete answer to this problem.

If you decide that your baby should sleep on his back, have him do so from the *very first night home.* If your baby is uncomfortable on his back, try the side. You may put a rolled-up towel under the baby's side for support. If your child continues to be uncomfortable, then, by all means, let the baby sleep on his stomach. After two or three months, he will make a decision on his own and do what feels best to *him*!

What about the bald spots on my baby's head?

Many parents complain about bald spots developing on the back of the baby's head from moving it from side to side while on her back, but the hair will eventually grow back and this should not be a great worry.

Does my baby dream?

Babies' sleep movements are similar to ours. They have what is called REM, or rapid eye movement sleep, as well as non-REM sleep.

During the period of REM sleep, it's almost like being able to watch a dream happening! She may make jerky or startled movements as she dreams, which is perfectly normal. Please don't panic!

Non-REM sleep on the other hand has several stages: 1) drowsiness; 2) light sleep; 3) deep sleep; and 4) very deep sleep. As the baby progresses from drowsiness to deep sleep, the breathing and all other activity will slow. In non-REM sleep, very little dreaming will occur.

The patterns of sleep will occur with relatively equal amounts of REM and non-REM sleep. As the baby gets older, the amount of REM or "dreaming" sleep will decrease and the sleep will become more relaxed.

Is it okay for the baby to sleep with me?

It is my feeling that, if you are comfortable having the baby sleep with you for the first few months of life and have developed some sort of pattern for doing this, then do so. However, after several months, certainly by one year (I prefer a younger age) your child needs a bed of his own. Make every effort to provide your child with some sort of bed away from you—if possible, in another room. You'll both need the rest and privacy at some point, and it's best to start as early as possible.

What's the best way to get my child to sleep?

The question of sleeping and just how to get a wide-awake child to sleep has puzzled parents and doctors alike, for years! Many, many methods have been tried: singing, rocking, walking and talking, swaddling, etc. All have worked at one time or another on all babies. The trick is to find one (or discover a new one) that works for *your* baby. Perhaps a few basic ideas can help:

- An hour or two before bedtime, reduce the amount of stimulation by turning off (or at least lowering the volume on) the TV or radio/stereo.

- RELAX, YOURSELF! If you are anxious about getting the baby to sleep, I guarantee the baby will sense it.

- Make sure the baby is warm and dry—not over- or underdressed and not hungry!

- See that nothing around or near him may be hindering his sleep. (Toys in the crib, etc.)

- Experiment with a night-light.

- GIVE HIM TIME! ninety-nine percent of babies will eventually adopt a reasonable sleep pattern—usually by about the fourth month.

- However tempting, sedating your baby (giving him medication to sleep) is *NOT* recommended!

Crying

It's a fact of life: ALL BABIES CRY! It is their only way of communicating and most use this particular tool with maddening regularity! However, as you get to know your baby, you'll begin to understand what he or she is trying to "tell" you with their special "language." She may be hungry, tired, uncomfortable, or she may simply want physical contact, a loving touch. Crying changes with age, understanding, and the maturity of your infant.

Try some of the things listed below to soothe your crying or cranky baby, and seek help from a friend or family member when you need to. I have never found a mother who was able to control ALL the crying, all by herself!

- Offer her something to eat—bottle or breast. Hunger is most often the cause of her irritability.

- Try the rocking chair—babies love the rhythm.

- Make sure the diaper is clean and dry. She may be wet or about to have a bowel movement.

- If you see that she has a diaper rash, leave the diaper off for a while. The fresh air will feel good and help to heal the rash.

- Moms that are breast-feeding need to watch their diet. Certain things that moms eat, like chocolate, can be upsetting to your baby's system.

- If you're bottle-feeding, ask about switching formulas. The one you're using may be upsetting her digestive system or she may not like the taste.

- Carry your baby around in a carrier you wear in the front of your body. Your movements and heartbeat will calm her.

- Take her for a ride in your car—strapped in the back seat in her car seat, of course!

- Try walking around outside for a change of scenery and fresh air.

- Cuddle her.

- Put her back in her crib and let her cry for a while. Check on her every few minutes. Some babies just *need* to be left alone to cry before sleep.

- HAVE PATIENCE!

Remember, as your baby ages, the crying will more likely be for specific reasons and require less guesswork on your part.

My mother says that if I pick the baby up every time he cries I'll spoil him rotten. Is this true?

Personally, I do not believe that an infant CAN be spoiled! Babies this age are simply not *smart* enough (mature enough) to distinguish between what they *want* and what they *need*. If your child is crying, he needs something; quite possibly (aside from being hungry or wet) what he needs is physical contact with someone who loves him! His developing brain, at this stage of life, simply cannot process the concept of "I want, therefore I'll cry, and *get* what I want!"

If you do not respond to your baby's needs, you are teaching him only that he must cry all the harder to get some sort of response. This is nerve-wracking to any parent. The child only becomes more and more demanding because his needs, whatever they are, are not being met. Everyone in the family is now anxious, tired, and frustrated because someone has suggested to them that to pick up a crying baby will "spoil him"!

Use your instincts. Hold and cuddle your baby. Let him know you'll be there for him. Everyone will be more content—the baby, because he will have the physical contact he needs; you, because the child will respond to the attention in a very positive manner—he'll stop crying! The crying will stop, not because he thinks he's won some sort of victory or manipulated you some-how—again, he's intellectually not capable of that level of cun-ning! His tears will stop because someone has cared enough to respond to a child who can express his needs only by crying! He needs (and will *later* discover that he also *wants*) physical contact with people who love him!

Stimulation

I must tell you that stimulation, physical and mental, and positive encouragement of your baby are extremely important, as the nature and amount of stimulation appears to influence his I.Q. Your willingness to do this will aid him as he develops men-tally and he will be more likely to handle future problems in a positive manner. Stimulation can be done in many ways—touch-ing, feeling, exploration, experimentation, etc.

Stimulation is necessary and the needs related to it are cru-cial. Your baby thrives on it. However, in your efforts to have your child learn *everything*, it's important that you know when to slow down! Your baby will let you know when he's had enough stimulation by being very tired and irritable!

Some of the things you can do to stimulate your baby:

◑ Pick up the baby. YOU WON'T SPOIL HIM!

◑ Talk to your child frequently.

◑ Touch and stroke your baby often.

◑ READ TO YOUR BABY, *DAILY*!

◑ Comfort (do not criticize!) your baby if he fails at something.

◑ *Praise* him when everything works!

◑ Kiss your baby often.

◑ Provide visual stimulation (mobiles, mirrors attached to the crib, etc.).

◑ Read, sing to him, and play music softly.

◑ Take him outside and identify the things he can see.

◑ Let him be with other adults and children.

Babyproofing the House

Just as with your automobile, the house must be made into a safe environment for your baby. In babyproofing your home for the new baby, you should be particularly cautious. Babies tend to get into, on, and under places you've probably considered *impossible* even for such a small person!

By the time your baby is six months old, you should have your home ready for her explorations. Place yourself in the position of your baby. *Get down on the floor and crawl around!* You may feel ridiculous, but you'll also discover why your home may look so interesting to a child!

What sorts of things should I be aware of?

- All electrical outlets—cover them, or get sockets that would be hard for a child to pull the cord out of or stick things in.

- Liquids under the sink—lock them up.

- Any poisons or hazardous materials in the house—get rid of them!

- Medicines—all should have childproof caps and be placed under lock and key.

- Block off all stairs and steps with baby gates to prevent falls.

- Shorten venetian blind cords (so that they are completely out of your baby's reach) and cover the ends with safety tassels to prevent entanglement and choking by the cord.

- Get rid of poisonous plants, such as poinsettia, ivy, elephant ear, etc.

- Check oven and refrigerator doors to make sure they close firmly and require more than a child's strength to open.

- Check chair and table legs for weakness; make sure they are sturdy and won't collapse.

- Check the opening and closing of doors—little bodies can easily be caught and seriously injured by doors that open and close too quickly.

- Check windows—all should have safety locks.

- Drawers should have locks when necessary.

- Make sure there are no small objects lying around, especially at lower levels where baby could reach.

- Have safety latches on all kitchen cabinets.

- Keep nonslip rugs and mats in all rooms—not just the bathroom.

- Have your water heater set at no higher than 120 degrees Fahrenheit.

- Pots and pans on the stove should have handles facing *away* from the edge.

- There should be no stools or steps that would allow a curious child an opportunity to crawl up and fall, or to reach things that may hurt her.

- Keep your baby in flame-retardant clothing as much as possible.

- The baby's room and furniture should be painted with **lead-free paint!**

- Pacifiers should not be attached to the baby's clothing if the child has to be left unattended for even a moment—any string that is used should be no longer than 3 inches.

- No sharp corners on furniture—pad them.

- Smoke alarms in every room.

- High chairs should be pushed away from counter tops where baby can reach things.

- Have a monitor in the nursery if possible.

- Keep crib away from windows, curtains, and cords.

- Keep all toiletries out of reach.

This list may seem long and complicated, and I'm sure that you have come up with some dos and don'ts of your own, but remember that you can NEVER be too careful! The best rule, always, is to *NEVER LEAVE YOUR BABY ALONE!*

Traveling with Baby

Traveling with your child can be an adventure or a nightmare! Again, the key phrase is "BE PREPARED!"

What sorts of things will we need when traveling?

- Travel with at least two small, soft washcloths and a towel or diaper for your shoulder for burps and spit-ups

- An adequate number of diapers for the length of time you will be out

- An extra baby blanket
- Adequate formula if you choose not to breast feed when traveling
- Change of clothing
- Sunscreen if you are going to have the baby outside
- Moist towelettes (baby wipes) for *parent's* hands—I do not recommend them for the baby's sensitive skin
- Large towel or pad for changing
- Travel sizes of powder, lotions, etc.
- Acetaminophen for infants
- Bibs
- Toys
- Pacifier
- After four months of age, a jar of unopened baby food and a spoon
- Plastic bags for soiled clothing, dirty utensils, unused food, dirty diapers, etc.

What should be in a "first aid kit" for the baby?

The following items should come in handy at one time or another:

- Nasal aspirator
- Calamine lotion
- Ear syringe
- Diaper rash ointment/zinc oxide
- Baby medicine dropper
- Cotton balls
- Rubbing alcohol
- Blanket
- Petroleum jelly/Vaseline®
- Flashlight
- Rehydration solution
- Paper cups

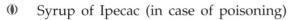

◑   Syrup of Ipecac (in case of poisoning)

◑   Adhesive bandages ½–1 inch

◑   Normal saline nose drops

◑   Scissors/blunt tip

◑   Hydrogen peroxide

◑   Gauze/roller, 1 inch, 2 inch

◑   Acetaminophen/drops or liquid *

◑   2-x-2– or 4-x-4 inch sterile dressing

◑   Infant ibuprofen/drops/liquid *

◑   Nail clippers

◑   Tweezers

◑   Soap

◑   Soft washcloths and hand towel

* Remember, infant drops are concentrated; read the label and always, if confused over the dose, speak to your baby's doctor.

Day Care and Nurseries

Children are much stronger and resilient than we give them credit for. They adapt to almost any situation or circumstance that is loving and caring. And so often in today's busy society we are reminded of the fact that our children *need* to become comfortable with other people so that they can adjust themselves to our not being around twenty-four hours a day every day.

The first step in accomplishing this is to be relaxed ourselves about choosing alternate caregivers for our children.

My mother says she will take care of the baby. I don't have any problem!

Don't be too sure! Though Grandma is the most obvious choice (after all, she did a great job with *you*!) it's very easy for friends and relatives to feel taken advantage of should, 1) your job hours change; 2) you make it *absolutely clear* when you will and will *not* need her; or, 3) you feel compelled to call upon her for babysitting chores other than during your working hours. ("Mom, could you keep the baby while I go shopping?"; "Mom, we want to go to a party, could you stay with the baby?"; etc.; etc.!)

But I'm not sure about day-care centers. How do I know they will take care of my baby the right way?

(The *right* way being *your* way, of course!) Obviously, nobody is going to care for your child the way you do. You're her mother and you know her best. You know when she's happy or sad; hungry or wet; sick or just irritable. You *know* you'll be there to pick her up when she needs you—you *don't* know if that person in the day care center will even *notice* her!

Parents have all sorts of *valid* concerns when considering placing their children in day care:

◑   Will she be fed when she's hungry?

◑   Will someone talk to her when she needs company?

◑   Will she get her share of toys and will they be clean?

◑   Will she be given the wrong formula or the wrong medication?

◑   Will the center call if there's a problem?

◑   Will her diaper be changed when she's wet?

◑   Will someone steal her clothes or lose her toys?

◑   Will they let someone take her out of the center without my consent?

◑   Is she happy, or does she cry all day?

The list is endless regarding the care of your child—and it should be. You should be absolutely confident and relaxed about the person(s) taking care of your baby while you're away. The only way is to rely on, first of all, your *instincts*. Next, talk to other parents with children in the center you're considering. If you hear negative comments or you just have a *feeling* it's not right—look elsewhere!

I realize that this particular advice is easier said than done. There are relatively few day care centers and even fewer that would measure up to our own standards. However, if you choose wisely, there will be little cause for concern.

What are some of the things I should ask or know about an alternate caregiver or day-care center for my child?

If you need an alternate caregiver or day-care center for your child, know the following information:

One Person: Your Home or Theirs:

1. Name, address, phone number, age?
2. Do they have a driver's license and car, or will they rely on other transportation?
3. What type of training, education, and/or certification do they have?
4. Do they have CPR training?
5. How flexible are they with their hours?
6. Do they cook or do housework?
7. How are they dressed? (Clean and neat?)
8. What are their salary requirements/benefits?
9. How do they discipline children?
10. What would they do with a crying, sick, or perhaps physically or mentally challenged infant?
11. Do they smoke?
12. How do they react to the child?
13. Does the child like them?

A Group of People—Day-Care Center:

1. Name, address, phone number of facility?
2. Ratio of caregivers to children—how many people are in charge of how many children?
3. Are they a licensed center and are the caregivers experienced, licensed day care workers?
4. What are the hours of operation and when are they closed?
5. What is the cost and how do they wish to be paid?
6. How many children are enrolled?
7. What is the overall quality of the center?

    a) eating facilities

    b) play facilities

    c) sleeping facilities

  8. What is the policy on caring for sick children?

  9. What is the policy on after-hours care and what is the cost?

10. Am I able to "drop in" at any time?

11. What is the center's reaction to my child?

12. What is my child's reaction to the center and the workers?

   If you are able to obtain satisfactory answers to these questions and any others that may occur to you, you can be reasonably sure that your baby will be well taken care of in your absence!

Chapter 4

Your Growing Baby

Baby's First Year

Regularly scheduled visits to your pediatrician, especially throughout your baby's first year of life, are an excellent way to help monitor your baby's growth and progress as well as keep an eye on her overall health. She will be growing by leaps and bounds—both physically and emotionally—and it's important to respond appropriately to each new stage of her development.

Are there general guidelines for when to bring my baby to the doctor?

During your baby's first year, you'll spend a lot of time talking with your pediatrician—in his office for scheduled health assessment visits, and on the phone when you have questions and/or emergencies between regular visits. Hopefully, you will have already become familiar with your doctor, before your child was born, during prenatal visits, which were discussed in chapter 1.

After your baby is born, your doctor will see both of you in the hospital, then schedule the regular series of office visits as recommended by the American Academy of Pediatrics. It will be up to you, as the baby's parents, to see that you keep these

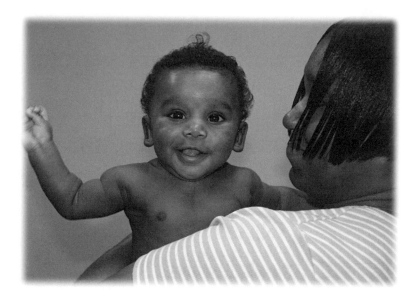

appointments. It's important for the health and overall development of your child that your doctor checks her periodically to make sure she's healthy and that she's developing normally. Usually, visits are scheduled at two to four weeks; two months; four months; six months; nine months; and twelve months. Your baby will grow rapidly during this first year, and the office visits will give you the opportunity to have documentation of these important milestones in your child's life. We will go into more detail about the physical examination in a separate chapter.

Approximately how quickly WILL my baby's weight and height change?

The weight and height of an infant are measured in direct proportion to nutrition and the natural growth of your baby. In the first few days of life, there is about a 10 percent weight loss as a result of the passage of the meconium stools we talked about in chapter 2, as well as the limited milk intake of the infant. After the first two weeks, most healthy babies will have regained their birth weight and will continue to gain from there.

The average baby will gain approximately two pounds per month during the first three months. Usually, the baby has *doubled* its birth weight by six months. At six months, the weight gain will drop normally to about one pound per month. At the end of one year, most babies will have tripled their birth weight.

Growth charts have been devised which reflect the growth of the majority of infants and children in the United States. Your pediatrician will plot the height, weight, and head circumference of your child during the first year. Deviation from normal standards will alert your pediatrician as to problems or potential problems that may be developing related to these growth measurements.

What is an AVERAGE weight gain during the first year?

The average weight of babies in the first year of life are as follows:

Boy's Weight	Age	Girl's Weight
7.5 lbs.	Birth	7.4 lbs.
13 lbs.	3 months	13 lbs.
19 lbs.	6 months	16 lbs.
23 lbs.	9 months	19 lbs.
25 lbs.	12 months	22 lbs.

What can I expect during my baby's FIRST MONTH?

During the first few weeks, your new baby will be eating, sleeping, and crying—and not much else! When awake, she may not seem very alert. Because of *your* emotional and physical exhaustion, this may be a mixed blessing! However, soon she'll begin to have longer periods when her eyes will open wide and she'll begin to notice her surroundings. She'll be able to focus on objects placed in her field of vision and will watch your face intently. She'll develop a strong grasping reflex (refer to chapter 2) and will be able to see black and white patterns. Your baby will also be able to focus and follow an object from the side to the front.

Your baby will also begin cooing, gurgling, and grunting and will respond to loud noises—some will respond to their parents' voices. She will turn her head when on her back or stomach and may even lift her head briefly from a flat surface.

The baby will also begin to develop a sense of trust—that she will be fed and comforted—and will feel gratification when these needs are met.

Nothing a new baby does elicits such excitement on the part of the parents as her first smile, which usually occurs when she's sleeping. However, one day, around the end of the first month, your baby will wake, look at *you*, and smile that wonderful, toothless grin!

This is also the first time both you and your new baby will visit the pediatrician's office. You should be familiar with your doctor by this time and feel at ease in talking with him about your concerns and the health of your child. However, no matter how prepared you think you may be for this visit, there are always things you have not anticipated! It's helpful at this point to have a list of questions—*written down*—to ask your doctor at this first visit.

What will happen during this two to four WEEK visit?

Your doctor will do a very thorough physical examination of your baby and inform you of the results—of both the current examination and the screenings done on your child while still in the hospital (see page 68 for a more thorough description of your baby's first physical examination). He will also tell you about the importance of immunizing your child and give you a schedule for immunizations—shots that will make your baby more resistant to some diseases.

Immunizations provide protection against targeted diseases. This is especially important as our society becomes increasingly mobile—relocating families to different areas of the country and world more and more frequently. The larger the group of people protected against a particular disease, the fewer the number of people who will have the disease. With adequate immunization, starting with an individual child, the disease will eventually disappear. (See page 78 for specific information about immunizations.)

Remember, your pediatrician is there to answer any questions you may have and to help you resolve any problems you may be having with the physical aspect of caring for your child—feeding, bathing, how to recognize signs of illness, etc.

Additionally, because this first month is likely to be very hectic and confusing for new parents, he'll discuss a number of emotional issues and offer advice on how to cope effectively with the challenges a new baby brings to all families!

What sorts of things will we talk about?

Because the well-being of your baby depends not only on the loving *physical* care he receives, your doctor will be interested in your *attitude* toward your baby.

- What type of personality does your baby appear to have—calm, active, or fussy—and how do you respond?
- What sort of sleep pattern, if any, has been established and how are you using it to your benefit?
- Are you receiving help with the baby? Is Dad helping? Are you asking your mother, grandmother, or close friend to help you with the baby?
- Are you and your partner, or you with your friends, able to spend some time away from the pressures of caring for the baby?
- Are you feeling overwhelmed or depressed?

These questions will reappear—with variations—during each office visit.

What can I expect during the SECOND MONTH?

By the time your baby is two months old, he will have begun to develop a personality and you'll more than likely see more smiles! He will be spending quite a lot of time studying his own hands and he'll begin to lose that grasping reflex. Though he'll be unable to control the movements of his hands at this point, he'll begin "batting" at objects placed near him. He'll hold his head up for longer periods of time and begin to notice the things and people around him—locating sounds and studying faces. He may also turn or roll from side to back.

You may also begin to distinguish different emotions and moods in your baby—whether he's happy or uncomfortable, for example.

I know the baby is scheduled for her second visit to the doctor during this month. What will happen this time?

As with each visit to your pediatrician, the baby will be examined thoroughly and her growth plotted on a chart for you.

You will receive instructions on how to read this chart and may be given a copy so that you'll be able to monitor your baby's progress between visits. Again, have your questions ready! By this visit, you will have had more time to get to know your baby and, since she is growing and changing every day, a whole new set of problems and/or concerns will likely have presented themselves since the last time you saw the doctor!

What will my child be like at THREE MONTHS?

By the third month, she'll have full neck control and be able to hold her head up for a full minute or two when she's on her stomach. She can hold objects and bring her hands up to her mouth. She may also push her head and shoulders up when on her stomach.

At three months, your baby will be a lot more social and begin to enjoy company, especially Mom and Dad! She'll wave her arms and stretch her legs and likely "talk" to anyone who'll listen, smile, and respond to her. She'll probably cry less and stop crying when you enter the room.

Her vision will be steadily improving and now she'll be able to see colors and follow moving objects.

What about the FOURTH MONTH?

This is an important month for many babies; he'll learn to roll from his stomach to back or from his back to side—or vice versa! That means, unfortunately, that you'll need to be extra attentive, as he now can easily roll off of a bed or changing table.

In addition to rolling from stomach to back, he'll probably be able to hold his head steady when pulled to a sitting position. He will also support some weight on his feet when pulled to a standing position. He'll begin to suck his fingers, creating a lot of drooling.

The baby will continue to become sociable, smiling and occasionally laughing out loud, but will have learned to get attention by fussing!

He'll play with hand rattles and link the sounds with objects. Your baby will also begin to explore *your* body as you hold him.

During this month, some pre-language sounds are heard—mostly consonant sounds like *N, D, P,* and *B.*

I know there's a doctor visit this month. Will there be anything different from the last one?

This month's visit will follow the same general pattern as the other visits; a thorough examination followed by the immunizations due at four months. The pediatrician will question you about how the baby tolerated the last shots and advise you that the baby will probably have a sore leg or be somewhat subdued after the immunizations. He will also direct you on the proper use of acetaminophen for any discomfort.

In his discussion with you, the doctor will answer your questions and will want to know something about your baby's accomplishments since the last visit. You'll probably have a lot of things to tell him!

During this visit, your pediatrician will be concerned with your child's eating patterns; the amount of formula he consumes within a twenty-four hour period; and what plans you have for starting your child on solid foods. He'll also discuss the baby's sleeping patterns, how much and how long he's sleeping, etc.

Your doctor will also remind you how important it is to talk to your baby and cuddle him—and keep him safe. You'll need to be aware of the things around your house that may pose a potential threat to your baby, now that he's becoming more and more active.

What's the FIFTH MONTH like?

She's really getting active now! She's rolling from her stomach to her back—and back again; reaching for objects and holding them in one hand and then transferring them to the other. She'll sit, with a little help from you at first, and she may crawl by reaching forward with her arms and pulling herself up.

She'll recognize her name and thoroughly enjoy your company. She'll chuckle and laugh during play, but will become more demanding—enjoying attention and letting you know how she feels when that attention is directed away from her!

He's SIX MONTHS old now! What can I expect?

Okay, now we're getting somewhere! This is the month when the baby will be able, most likely, to sit up by himself by positioning his hands beside him. He'll need only a little help from you, but watch him carefully! He's still learning and growing and is not yet an expert at balancing; he can topple easily. Be sure he's on a soft surface. If you're holding him, he will enjoy jumping up and down.

At six months, your baby will start to imitate the sounds he hears and will become increasingly interested in new things around him. He'll also start to look for objects he has dropped.

He'll start to munch and chew—may begin teething—and play with his toes by sticking them in his mouth! Lots of things are starting to end up in his mouth now that his hand/eye co-ordination is improving!

Your little one is now becoming very attached to certain objects, food, and people, especially the people who take care of him. However, he will probably be content playing by himself for a while, but will reach out his arms to you with a happy smile when you get back to him!

The baby may not be quite ready to crawl, but he's starting to learn the basics. He'll push himself on his stomach, letting his arms move him along.

Another office visit is due this month. Anything new?

By this time, you're becoming an old pro at office visits with your growing baby. You and your doctor are very familiar with each other by now and both of you should be comfortable with questions and familiar with your baby's reactions to the visits. This visit may focus less on the physical changes and concentrate more on your child's activities, interaction with the environment, and motor skills development.

The doctor will also be interested in how your family is adjusting to the baby's schedules and the overall demands of being parents.

NOTE: Speak to your pediatrician if your baby, from three to six months, does *NOT*:

- Turn toward sound
- React to bright light
- Follow objects with eyes
- Smile
- Raise head while lying on stomach
- Roll over by five months

What happens during the SEVENTH MONTH?

During this month she will graduate from simply grasping objects to being able to hold something with her fingers for as long as she wants to. She is beginning to enjoy touching and feeling the objects within her reach, which may not be as limited as you think. She's sitting up well now and can scoot around on her bottom to get to where she wants to go!

The baby noises she's been making are beginning to turn into the sounds that will soon become actual words! Usually, these will be something like "ga-ga" or "ba-ba." NOTE: It is important that parents NOT talk "baby talk" to their increasingly vocal babies. Babies tend to imitate what they hear, and it's best that they hear our language as it should be spoken, though maybe at a slower speed, at first.

We have all noted variations in speech from one ethnic group to another, but overall, there is a common thread in the way all parents, mothers and fathers alike, speak to infants; it's what is called "Parentese."

Parentese—the way adults, especially mothers, talk to their children—is spoken in a higher than normal frequency, higher than normal pitch, but it's *talk*, and not "babble"!

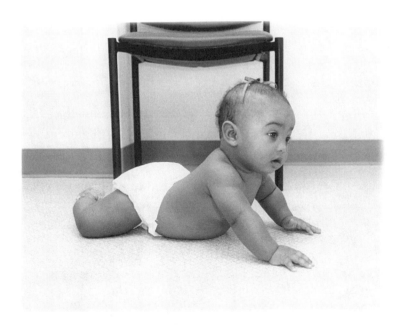

Talking to your baby, slowly and distinctly, from the very beginning of his life lays a foundation for learning later in life. Repetition of simple words and phrases and the expression on your face can communicate volumes to your child. Tell him about your day and what you're doing as you feed him or change his diaper—and smile!

She's already EIGHT MONTHS old! Will she be able to stand by herself?

It is during the eight month that your little one may really start moving! She'll begin by rocking back and forth on all fours and then dropping back to her stomach to move herself along. Her legs are still fairly weak, but she may be able to manage standing for a few moments while holding onto something.

This is also the month when she may start that exasperating habit of dropping things on the floor on purpose, just to see if someone will pick them up!

The NINTH MONTH has really brought some changes. What else can I expect?

Having some trouble feeding your child? He's asserting his independence now and learning that he has some degree of control over a spoon, bowl, or cup. This can be very messy for everyone and extremely frustrating to you; there's food everywhere! However, it is important that you let him do as much as he can by himself! Having some control over his life is as important to him as it is to you.

Usually, this is the month when the word "NO" is seemingly the only thing he hears! Of course, we *must* say "no" at times in order to keep our children out of danger, and he will soon learn what he may and may not do.

The baby can now sit alone and pull himself up to a standing position. The legs are getting stronger every day! Your baby may stand up and attempt to move or walk sideways. He will do this while holding onto something for support. This is the time when babyproofing your house will begin to pay off!

He is still sociable, but is now wary of strangers and will likely stay in close proximity to Mom or Dad when visited by someone he does not know.

What will the nine month office visit be like?

This visit may be a bit more traumatic than the others simply because your child is growing quickly, becoming more aware of things around him, and consequently, more fearful of strangers and strange places. He can now, because of his growing awareness, remember, for instance, that the doctor's office is where he was stuck with that needle! You may have to hold him in your lap for part of the examination.

After another thorough physical examination, your doctor will discuss your child's responsiveness: smiling, playing with toys, finger-feeding, grasping, sitting, etc. He will also want to know how much you think your baby understands when you talk to him—and if he attempts to "talk" back to you.

Again, have your questions ready. All sorts of issues—separation, baby-sitters, day care, teething, safety—may be a part of your discussion during this visit.

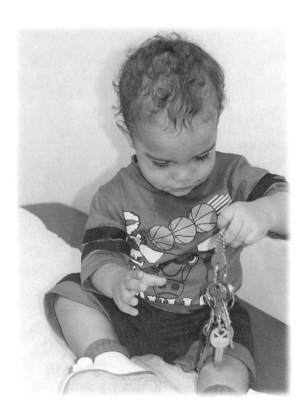

My child is TEN MONTHS old now and is beginning to try to walk—but not quite making it!

She will slide her feet, placing them flat on the floor using her hands only for balance. Next, she'll be able to pick her feet up and step, using a hand-over-hand motion. When she can close the gap between pieces of furniture, she'll be very close to actually walking. And talking isn't too far away. The "da-da's" and the "ma-ma's" will begin to *mean* something to all of you!

NOTE: Speak to your pediatrician if your six to ten month-old:

◉   Does not "talk" to you, repeating syllables by nine months

◉   Does not reach for objects or is unable to grasp objects by nine months

◉   Cannot stand with support by ten months

◉   Does not distinguish the familiar from unfamiliar (people) by ten months.

We're in the ELEVENTH MONTH, and things are moving very quickly!

Though I believe children should be read to from birth, you *definitely* should have begun by now. This practice may well instill a lifelong desire for learning! Just speak slowly and carefully and she'll soon begin to imitate these sounds and words. And remember: "Parentese" is fine; babble or baby talk is not!

She has become very mobile and is able to discover many strange and exciting things which delight her; however, she may be a little frightened by this independence and begin to want to be around you a little more often. Be sure to give her the attention she needs, but don't be afraid to leave her—she'll be fine once she discovers that nothing awful will happen when Mom leaves the room—and that you *will* eventually return!

She may begin to "creep" on hands and knees and can probably stand alone. She is probably drinking from a cup now. She can also move her little hands and fingers to get objects out of tight places.

It's been TWELVE MONTHS! A whole year! Where did the time go?

Your baby is about to celebrate his first year of life! It doesn't seem possible, does it? And just look at him! He's standing without support for short periods of time and is probably able to take a few steps, with or without your help. He is understanding more and more of what you say to him and you are beginning to understand *his* first words! Though he may love this new "walking and talking," he may do one or the other for a while with more concentration as he perfects his skill in both.

Remember that children learn by watching—and he's been paying quite close attention to you! He is starting to imitate your actions and the actions of others around him. He may try to do many of the things he sees you doing during your day: talking on a play phone; "loving" a favorite stuffed animal the way you hug *him*; trying to get his clothes over his head; trying to "write" by scribbling with a crayon; etc. From now on, the possibilities are endless as your baby starts to "grow up"!

He also is able to use a spoon with varying degrees of success!

This will be the last doctor visit for this year. Will there be any significant changes during the visit?

This is a milestone for everyone! It's been a whole year of learning and growing with your baby. You've learned to understand each other and adapt, somewhat, to each other's personalities and schedules. He's changed so much from the day you brought him home and he's changing rapidly each day—but you've changed, too. You've discovered that you're a lot more capable than you ever believed you could be!

The last doctor visit of your baby's first year will include a routine examination and the immunizations scheduled at this time.

Usually, around this time, punishment and setting limits become concerns, and your pediatrician may offer some advice on how to approach this sensitive subject. Your baby will likely seem to be everywhere at once, and into things that may harm him. You need to know how to deal with this by knowing how to help your child express joy, sadness, anger, fear, and frustration in a positive manner.

Overall, I am sure you new parent(s) have made it through this hectic, sometimes frustrating and frightening first year with flying colors! Just continue loving, cuddling, supporting, talking to, playing with, and enjoying your baby. The next year will bring new concerns and challenges, but none that you can't handle.

And as you watch your baby turn into a "real little person," I believe you'll consider it all worth the trouble!

First Physical Examination by the Pediatrician

Now let's backtrack a bit and go over the specifics of your baby's first visit to her doctor's office (between two and four weeks). At that time, a comprehensive examination will take place and the doctor will be available for any advice or counseling you may need.

Why types of questions should I ask my doctor?

Again, you can help your doctor answer your questions by being prepared—write your questions down beforehand if you need to.

You need to know whether your baby's weight, height, length, and head size fall within a normal range and if the baby is developing normally. While your baby may or may not deviate from these "normals," your doctor will take into account your genetics, any illness of the baby, whether term or premature, and your infant's birth weight in discussing these important components of your baby's growth.

◑   Ask about the baby's vision and hearing.

◑   Ask about the results of the PKU and thyroid and sickle-cell anemia screening (see page 23).

◑   Ask about any problems as a result of the exam.

◑   Ask what to expect in the next few months concerning your baby's overall development. (You may find I have already answered some of your questions in this section of the book.)

◑   Ask for a permanent health record to record your baby's progress and to keep a record of immunizations (shots).

◑   Write down any problems or questions for the next visit!

Your physician will be very thorough with this important, first examination. Here are the major things he'll be checking:

What should my baby weigh?

Your baby will be weighed on a "baby scale" and only clothed in a diaper. The weight is taken and plotted on a graph, much like the ones on pages 70 and 71. Your baby's length will also be measured (from the top of the head to the soles of her feet) and entered on the graph. Your baby's combined measurements will help the doctor determine if your baby falls within normal range by comparing them to national percentiles (as seen on the graphs for boys on pages 70 and 71). When infants have measurements that are above the ninety-seventh percentile or below the third percentile, they will require more evaluation, as will infants whose height and weight are different by more than two percentile lines or categories.

What are fontanels?

Your pediatrician will examine your baby's head to feel specifically for soft areas called fontanels. There are usually two major fontanels: anterior—located in the front of the skull; and posterior—located at the rear of the skull. If you run your finger down the suture line of the skull (the middle of the skull, front to back), you will feel these "open" spaces. The posterior fontanel is open and may remain so for as long as eighteen months. The anterior usually closes by six months. These soft openings allow for growth and make it possible for the skull to accommodate the growing brain.

What causes molding, lumps, and bumps?

If your baby has a lump on his head, he probably had a fairly rough passage as he was "getting born"! This may happen as a result of the baby's head hitting the wall of the vagina, causing some bleeding under the infant's scalp. These lumps are usually limited to the specific areas of the skull next to the sutures and are called cephalhematomas. These will go away after the first two or three months and do not pose any long-term problems.

Another lump that you may see is a result of fluids present in the soft tissue of the brain. This may be because the baby's head was held in one position inside the vagina for several hours during birth. In medical terminology, it is called a caput succedaneum, which is Latin for "conehead." This usually disappears within a few days after birth.

The baby's head could be odd-shaped because of the overlap of the sutures while the infant is inside of the mother's body. This is called molding and probably won't be noticeable after about three days.

Boys: Birth to 36 Months Physical Growth
National Center for Health Statistics Percentiles

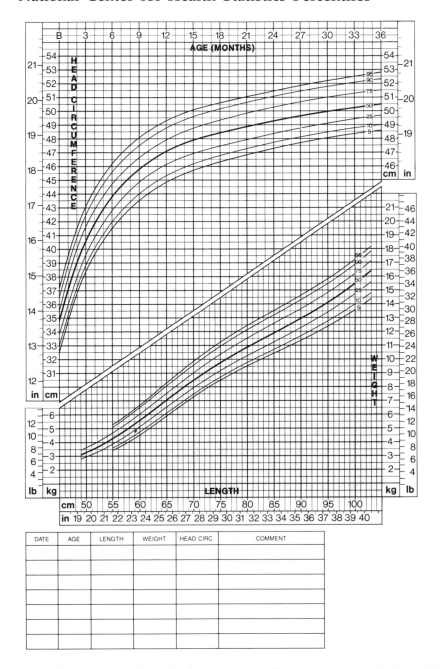

DATE	AGE	LENGTH	WEIGHT	HEAD CIRC.	COMMENT

Used with permission of Ross Products Division, Abbott Laboratories, Columbus, OH 43216 From NCHS Growth Chts. © 1982 Ross Products Division, Abbott Laboratories

Girls: Birth to 36 Months Physical Growth
National Center for Health Statistics Percentiles

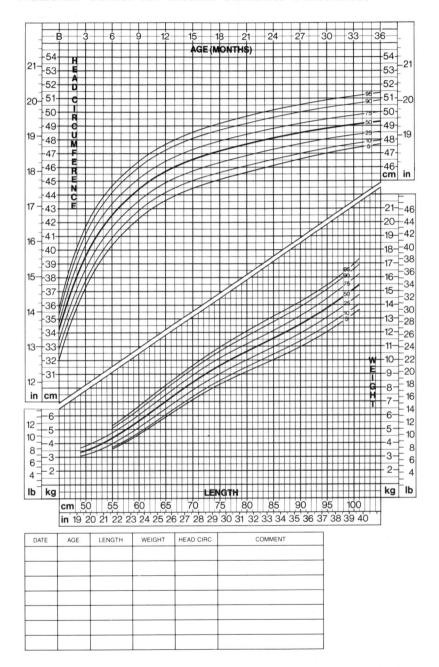

DATE	AGE	LENGTH	WEIGHT	HEAD CIRC.	COMMENT

Used with permission of Ross Products Division, Abbott Laboratories, Columbus, OH 43216 From NCHS Growth Chts. © 1982 Ross Products Division, Abbott Laboratories

Why does he check the size of my baby's head?

The size of your baby's head is very important to your pediatrician. The doctor or nurse will put a tape measure around
the head at the longest area—front to back—and take three measurements—recording the longest value on a graph (see page 70).
The measurements will give the doctor an indication as to
whether the head or brain is of normal size. He will also be able
to tell whether the head grew too quickly or too slowly, and will
be able to monitor this information on a table with a column for
head size (see page 70). Generally, boys will have slightly larger
heads than girls. Racially, there appears to be no difference noted
in head sizes nor does intellectual ability appear to be determined
by head size. The average measurements of head size (in centi-
meters and inches) during the first year are:

Age	Centimeters	Inches
Birth	35	14
2 months	40	16
6 months	44	17
9 months	45	18
12 months	49	19

See graph page 70.

We expect a big baby to have a bigger head than a small
baby, and some families, because of genetics, will have babies
with large heads.

Your doctor will measure your baby's head and compare it
to the baby's age and weight. If the head is too large or too small
for age and weight, the baby will be followed closely for any
evidence of present or developing abnormality.

Explain the examination of my baby's eyes.

The color, size, and shape of your baby's eyes are checked
by your pediatrician on the initial visit. When your doctor looks
at the eyes, he examines them for symmetry and response.

Symmetry refers to whether the eyes are located in the same
plane, i.e., the same line. Response refers to whether the pupils
are the same size and if they open and close in response to light.

The doctor will check the eyelids and the position of the
eyes in their sockets. He will use a light to examine the surface

of the eyeball. He will also note the movement of the eyes with and without a light.

He will examine the eyes internally with an instrument called an ophthalmoscope, looking for a reflection of light from the eye back to the instrument, and to check for any abnormalities present.

Many babies appear to be cross-eyed due to weak eye muscles. Most often, these muscles will become strong and the appearance will be normal in about six months. If the condition has not improved by this time, you may be referred to a pediatric eye specialist for further tests.

Some babies will seem to have much more tearing in one eye or another, which is usually due to blocked tear ducts. Most of the time, this condition will correct itself, but sometimes the tear duct may need to be massaged. This will be demonstrated by your doctor. If the tearing condition does not correct itself within six or eight months, your doctor will probably refer you to a pediatric ophthalmologist. Some babies may have a thick, cruddy discharge from their eyes. This may be normal, but could possibly be an infection acquired while coming through the birth canal—you should have this checked by your doctor.

Can my baby see when she's born?

Unless there is some visual defect which can be determined by your pediatrician, the answer is YES, your baby can see at birth! The baby's vision may not be what you expect, but this will improve as she ages. At birth, the baby may be able to see a distance of between eight and fifteen inches in front of her face.

Explain the examination of my baby's mouth.

Your doctor will be looking for deformity and asymmetry—when the two sides are abnormally uneven. After examining the lips, the doctor will use a tongue depressor to observe the gums and inner lining of the mouth, called the mucous membrane. He notes the color of the gums and the lining of the mouth and looks for the presence of any growths. The palate, which is located at the top or "roof" of the mouth, is checked, along with the uvula, the little bit of tissue hanging down at the back of the mouth.

Occasionally, you will see some small, white lumps called Epstein's pearls which have no known function! They'll disappear within a few months.

Why does he examine the baby's neck?

When your doctor examines the neck, he will sometimes find a lump. This may have resulted from forceps used when the baby was delivered, which in turn caused some bleeding down the muscle inside the neck. The body will usually take care of this without any medical intervention.

He will also feel the thyroid gland to check for enlargement, as well as to note the location of the windpipe to make sure it is in the middle of the throat. The neck will also be checked for "range of motion." As noted earlier, sometimes your baby will get an infusion of blood in the muscle along the neck, causing the muscle to contract. A condition called "head tilt" may result. Most babies with head tilt can be treated by simply stretching the muscle. If you note a lump in the neck and/or your baby has a head tilt, please make sure that you notify your doctor. With stretching, it will usually take several months to show improvement.

What is he looking for when checking the chest?

The chest is checked for symmetry and any abnormal masses or growths. In many infants, the breast buds may be prominent. This is usually due to hormone transfer from the mother to the child. With time and removal of the hormone influence in the body, the prominence of the breasts will reduce to a more normal appearance. Sometimes, the breasts will weep a white discharge as a result of this hormone transfer, but this will soon stop.

As if these peculiar-sounding things weren't enough, an occasional infant will have what is called an "accessory nipple"! This is usually seen as a darker area below the breast. While of no significance in the majority of cases, they have been rarely associated with the presence of renal (kidney) problems, especially if the baby is born with *other* signs of defects or abnormalities, called congenital abnormalities.

What does he look for while examining the lungs?

In the newborn period, your baby may breathe at a rate of between fifty and sixty breaths per minute. After the first three weeks to a month, that rate usually drops to between thirty and forty breaths per minute.

The doctor will listen for abnormal sounds in the lungs that would indicate some respiratory problem at birth. In the vast majority of children, this examination is negative.

If your pediatrician notes any problem, it most likely will be rapid breathing; the baby's stomach will be moving rapidly and she may be gasping for breath. If this situation occurs while the baby is still in the hospital, an assessment can be done to evaluate the cause.

If you are already home, watch for rapid breathing, wheezing, or unusual noises. Usually, babies with respiratory problems will exhibit these symptoms. In addition, they may also have blue fingers and toenails and will flare their nostrils. At any rate, if you notice any of these things, call your pediatrician immediately—he will advise you.

What makes the baby's stomach look so big?

The baby's abdomen often appears very full-looking and big. This is perfectly normal. In fact, the abdomen on most babies will seem large until the child reaches about three years of age. In the newborn period, the abdomen is large because of the large liver and the expansion of the lungs with the downward pushing of the diaphragm. The stomach lies in a horizontal position in the abdomen during infancy and becomes more vertical during childhood. Over the first year, the capacity of the stomach increases dramatically.

There may be a small "line" noted, in most African American babies, down the center of the abdomen from the cord to the pubic bone—it probably reflects the closure of the lower abdomen in utero. This line will disappear by the time the baby is a year old.

On examination, your doctor is looking for any large masses or structures which do not appear to be in the appropriate places. These organs/structures in the abdomen may include the liver, spleen, stomach, kidneys, and intestinal tract. The umbilical cord usually has fallen off by the time of this visit. The navel area will be checked to see that the stump has healed properly and if an umbilical hernia is present.

The umbilical hernia opening is a small hole in the abdomen covered by skin. It is due to a weakness in the anterior stomach wall. Normal muscle and tissue reinforcement did not take place properly. As a result you may see the protrusion with only air present or in some cases stomach contents (usually intestines) may spill over. In the vast majority of cases this poses no problem and if they appear stuck the contents can be pushed back or, more often, ignored. As stated earlier, most of the time only air come through the small hole. In those cases where the opening is large, or there is pain, or the stomach contents get trapped, surgery is indicated. Most hernias "go away" as the child ages. The hole closes, the skin no longer protrudes. A good rule is if it is not bothering your child—leave it alone.

Umbilical hernias occur more commonly in African American infants (32 percent) versus Caucasian infants (4 percent).

How does he examine the heart?

When examining the heart, the first thing your pediatrician will do is use his fingertips to feel the chest wall to detect any unusual rumbles. He will also check the pulses as part of the cardiovascular examination, both at the wrist and in the inguinal (groin) area. He will also check to see how fast or slow, regular or irregular, the heart is beating. His stethoscope will alert him to both normal and abnormal heart sounds.

In the newborn, it is not uncommon to detect a heart murmur. Heart murmurs are sounds that are made by the blood flowing through the valves of the heart or within the heart. In some newborns, one of the vessels leading to the heart may not close as rapidly as it should and will result in a loud heart murmur. This vessel is usually the one called a patent ductus arteriosus (PDA). The majority of PDAs will spontaneously close, i.e., close by themselves without medical intervention.

In most infants, the majority of heart murmurs are "innocent" murmurs and represent the normal flow of blood through the valves across the heart or through the heart.

The baby's heart seems to be beating so fast!

The newborn's heart rate varies from 95 to 150 beats per minute, but will beat slower as she gets older. In fact, in the newborn period, we consider rates less than 90 to be slow; greater than 160 as fast. When either end of the spectrum is reached, your doctor should investigate. During the first year, the heart rate changes to between 80 and 125 beats per minute.

Remember, your baby naturally has a rapid heart rate that will cause the heart to beat faster in order to provide appropriate circulatory functions.

What does the doctor do when he looks at my baby's sex organs?

You will notice that your baby's genital organs are rather large. This is normal during this time. Your doctor will look for any hernia in boys and girls. If your baby is a girl, he will make sure the vagina is normal looking. If your baby is a boy, he will make sure the penile opening is adequate and that the scrotum (sac) has two descended testes.

What else will he check?

Believe it or not, the hands of your baby will give the doctor an indication of any genetic problems. When examining the hands, he will look for any deformity or additional creases and folds. He will know whether or not the fingers are curved, clubbed, elongated, or are unusual in any way, which may indicate a genetic problem.

The legs and feet are carefully checked for length, as well as for signs of in-toeing or out-toeing, bowing or contracture; the hips for proper flexion, extension, and range of motion.

The tibia is the big bone in the lower leg. When it is not aligned properly, it will cause the foot to swing in, resulting in tibia torsion. Many babies are misdiagnosed as having an "in-toed" condition when, in reality, the problem is with their legs rather than their feet. Tibia torsion actually occurs in less than 5 percent of all babies and is not usually corrected until the child is between one and two years old.

What is meant by "flat feet"?

This is a normal occurrence in the infancy and toddler stages. You must be aware that the arch of the baby's foot is filled with *fat*, giving the impression of a flat foot. After about eighteen months, and your child has begun walking, your pediatrician can assess this situation more closely.

Immunizations

Having your baby immunized is one of the most essential and important things you can do for your child, especially if you live in a crowded environment. I say this because many people live in places where epidemics are more likely to occur—such as in public housing as opposed to single family dwellings.

No parent likes to see their baby in pain, but YOU MUST NOT IGNORE THE IMPORTANCE OF IMMUNIZATIONS! And believe me, the baby dislikes it every bit as much as you! The goal of immunization is the elimination of the disease involved. The major benefit to you of immunization is that your child is protected against that disease. As more and more people are immunized, the chances of your child catching that disease becomes less and eventually that disease will disappear requiring no immunization. The pinch or sting of an injection or the taste of an oral vaccine is over in a moment—the benefits last a lifetime.

There may be benefits, but I've heard that some vaccinations cause terrible side effects. Is this true?

Hearing that some vaccines cause some adverse side effects makes parents decidedly uncomfortable and unsure about whether or not the baby really *needs* this. But be assured, the risk is very small. Most of the side effects are minor; a soreness or a mild fever. Each year the vaccines are improved to reduce the side effects.

Your pediatrician is *required* to provide you with literature outlining the possible consequences of any immunizations your child receives.

What are the types of vaccines my baby will receive?

The following information will give you an idea of the types of immunizations required for your child and when they should be administered:

Hepatitis B: This condition is caused by a DNA virus and can be transmitted by contact with infected blood (as by a transfusion). When spread through the blood, hepatitis can cause any number of serious diseases, including acute hepatitis, liver disease, and cancer of the liver.

Three doses of the vaccine are necessary:

◑   Two vaccines between birth and 4 months

◑   One vaccine at 6 to 18 months

If your baby is not immunized against HBV when he's an infant, it definitely should be done by the time he is twelve years old.

Diphtheria, Tetanus, Pertussis (DPT or DTaP): Diphtheria is a respiratory disease spread by coughs and sneezes and can become so serious that it causes paralysis, heart failure, and finally suffocation.

Tetanus is a disease that cannot be passed from person-to-person, but usually enters the body through a cut or another type of wound. This bacteria produces poison that attacks the nervous system. Stepping on a rusty nail or an animal bite may lead to tetanus.

Pertussis, also known as whooping cough, can easily and quickly be spread through coughing and sneezing. Pertussis begins with cold-like symptoms, but turns into severe coughing spells. Babies under nine months of age are in particular danger because pertussis can cause pneumonia, convulsions, and encephalitis (an inflammation or infection of the brain).

Five doses of the DTaP vaccine are necessary *before* your child's sixth birthday:

◑ The first at 2 months

◑ The second at 4 months

◑ The third at 6 months

◑ The fourth at 12 to 18 months

◑ The fifth at 4 to 6 years

A tetanus/diphtheria (TD) booster shot is also required at eleven to sixteen years of age and every ten years after that. (Have you had *yours* lately?!)

Hemophilus Influenza—Type B: This vaccine is commonly referred to as HIB and is given to prevent several very serious conditions, including meningitis and pneumonia. Hemophilus influenza illness can be spread through the air by coughing, or by direct contact. Prior to the introduction of this vaccine in 1990, over 20,000 children a year contracted Hemophilus influenza type B meningitis. It was the most common cause of meningitis in the United States Other children, mostly under two years old, had many other serious infections. Since the introduction of the vaccine, invasive, serious Hemophilus influenza disease in young children has declined by 95 percent.

Four doses of HIB are given:

◑ The first at 2 months

◑ The second at 4 months

◑ The third at 6 months

◑ The fourth at 12 to 15 months

Polio: This is a viral disease causing severe muscle pain, difficulty in breathing, and paralysis in the arms and legs.

The Salk vaccine was introduced in 1955. Before that, over 18,000 cases of paralytic polio were reported during the epidemic years. Since the 1960s the incidence of polio has been steadily declining and has almost been entirely eliminated. There are fewer than five cases per year currently reported in the United States—thanks to the vaccine.

Four doses of the polio vaccine (IPV or OPV) are given usually at the same time we give the DTaP. Polio comes in an injected version (IPV) and an oral version (OPV). The following sequence is recommended at this time.

◑ The first at 2 months—IPV

◑ The second at 4 months—IPV

◑ The third at 6 to 18 months—OPV

◑ The fourth at 4 to 6 years (before school)—OPV

The IPV's strength is in not causing the spread of vaccine-associated paralytic polio (VAPP). Given the way currently recommended, we appear to get greater protection from epidemic polio and adequate defense against contracting VAAP.

Measles, Mumps, Rubella (MMR): Measles is a contagious disease spread through coughs and sneezes, and can cause serious secondary infections such as encephalitis and middle-ear infections.

Mumps is a viral infection that causes headaches, swollen glands, and fever.

Rubella, also known as German measles, is very contagious, but relatively mild, causing fever and a rash, but for a pregnant woman can be very serious. If the woman catches rubella early in her pregnancy, it can cause miscarriage or severe birth defects. In addition to preventing the disease, the vaccine is given in order to protect pregnant women from contracting rubella from an infected child.

Two MMR vaccines are necessary:

◑   The first at 12 to 15 months

◑   The second at either 4 to 6 years, or 11 to 12 years

Chicken Pox (or varicella): This disease like measles, is highly contagious and caused by a virus. It is spread through direct contact with an infected child. While there is a raised rash with measles, chicken pox will present itchy, blister-like, fluid-filled bumps that will dry up in three to five days and then scab over. Unfortunately, the child will be contagious one or two days *before* the rash appears and for as long as the scabs are visible on the body! It can also take from ten to twenty-one days for symptoms of headaches and fever to appear after the child has been exposed.

◑   One varicella vaccine is now recommended at *12 to 15 months of age.*

As I said, no one likes to get a shot; we don't even like to give them, but maybe these suggestions will make things a little easier for you and your child:

◑   Prepare your child ahead of time and NEVER *LIE* TO HER BY TELLING HER THAT IT WON'T HURT! If your child is old enough to understand what you are telling her, explain that she WILL feel a little sting, but that it will be over very quickly. Also, stress that the shot is necessary to keep her healthy.

◑   Stay calm yourself! Remember, your child is usually as anxious or as calm as *you* are!

◑   Try distracting your child as the injection is being given by talking to her—anything to keep her mind (and maybe yours!) off that needle!

◑   And please NEVER THREATEN A MISBEHAVING CHILD WITH, "IF YOU DON'T BE GOOD, YOU'RE GONNA GET A SHOT!" This is *guaranteed* to make her afraid, not only of injections, but of paying a visit to the doctor at all!
    DO NOT NEGLECT THIS IMPORTANT ASPECT OF CARING FOR YOUR CHILD! IT CAN POSSIBLY SAVE YOUR CHILD'S LIFE!

Recommended Schedule for Immunization of Infants and Children

Age	Vaccine
Birth	HPV
2 months	DTaP, HIB, IPV, HPV
4 months	DTaP, HIB, IPV
6 months	DTaP, HIB, HPV
12-15 months	DtaP, OPV, HIB, MMR, Var
4 years	DTaP, OPV, MMR
11-12 years	Td (Var, MMR, HBV if needed)

Vaccine abbreviations
HPV = Hepatitis B vaccine; DTaP = Diphtheria-Tetanus-Acellular Pertussis vaccine; HIB = Haemophilus influenzae type B vaccine; Td = Adult type Tetanus and Diphtheria vaccine; IPV = inactivated poliovirus vaccine; OPV = oral polio vaccine; MM = measles, mumps, rubella vaccine; Var = varicella vaccine.

Medical Concerns/Problems in Newborns

The most common medical problems found in newborns relate to respiratory distress, i.e., breathing disorders. These disorders range from no breathing at all to very labored or rapid breathing. Your pediatrician will consider problems related to breathing as a medical emergency.

My doctor says my baby did not get enough oxygen. What does he mean?

When the level of oxygen is low in the baby's circulation, the condition is called asphyxia. Your baby's blood levels become acidotic (low alkaline level), and there is a buildup of carbon dioxide. Asphyxia can be a result of problems prior to birth, such as a premature rupture of the placenta, or high blood pressure in the mother. After birth, when blood gases are measured, the baby is considered to be in distress when a low pH and a high carbon dioxide level, coupled with a low oxygen level, is found. These infants will have difficulty breathing and may require resuscitation. Mothers who are considered at high risk for having children with asphyxia are those with hypertension (high blood pressure), diabetes, or anemia. Post-mature or premature infants are also considered to be at risk.

What is TTN?

TTN (transient tachypnea of the newborn) is classified as a benign condition of rapid breathing. These infants may require some oxygen, but TTN usually resolves within three or four days.

My doctor says my baby is anemic. What does that mean?

When your child's red blood cell count is below normal, he is said to be anemic. In general, anemia is a result of inadequate production of red blood cells or the destruction of red blood cells. Anemia may be caused by infections that occurred while in the uterus, acute blood loss at birth (due to abruption—a placental accident—or some other physical incident), inherited diseases, or bone marrow problems (that lead to less than normal red cell production).

When an infant or child is anemic, he becomes lethargic, has little appetite, and does not grow normally. He can become anemic from decreased red cell production as well as inadequate iron in the diet, an essential component in the production of hemoglobin. Hemoglobin is the part of red cells that moves oxygen into the tissue and carries carbon dioxide out. Starting the baby on cow's milk too soon may decrease iron in your baby's system. Cow's milk contains very little absorbable iron and should not be given to children under one year of age. Cow's milk may also cause intestinal irritation and red blood cell loss.

When red cells are destroyed, it is called hemolysis. One of the more common hemolytic disorders is sickle-cell anemia (see page 23). Children and adults with hemolytic disorders can become profoundly anemic.

Your doctor will do tests to determine the cause of the anemia, if not readily apparent, and treat your child for the condition.

My baby was jittery. My doctor says his sugar was low. Is there a long-term problem?

Babies, after birth, sometimes cannot maintain their blood glucose (sugar) levels. Shortly after your infant is born, the nursery staff will obtain a glucose level. If your baby experiences jitters, poor appetite or feeding, was lethargic or had seizures, it becomes more urgent to check the sugar level. Low blood sugar is called hypoglycemia. Hypoglycemia also occurs frequently in infants of diabetic mothers and in post-mature and premature infants. Babies who have infections or asphyxia are also prone to be hypoglycemic. It is necessary to treat this condition quickly while looking for the cause of the problem.

Symptoms of hypoglycemia can be poor feeding, inactivity, jitteriness, poor cry, or even seizures. If this is the case with your baby, your pediatrician will treat the condition immediately. Once corrected, most babies maintain their own glucose levels within a normal range.

What is sepsis?

Babies who contract infections, either from viruses or bacteria in the blood stream, are said to have sepsis. The more serious infections seem to be bacterial, though some viral infections can be disastrous and can affect any organ. If your doctor suspects sepsis, he will discuss this with you and request permission to do some special tests in order to attempt to identify the organism, especially if it is bacterial. These tests may include a lumbar puncture (spinal tap), blood culture, and bladder tap. Your baby may be placed on antibiotics until the culture results are known. In the majority of cases, the cultures are negative and the antibiotics can be discontinued—assuming your baby appears improved—and the baby will be discharged home. If the cultures are positive, the causative organism is identified and treatment is continued for a specified period of time.

Sepsis is a life-threatening medical condition. If caught early, the majority of infants recover without any further complications or problems. The complications to sepsis may occur in relation to the type of organism and the time it takes to make a diagnosis and start treatment.

What are some of the common birth defects?

In 1 out of 500 infants born, there is a condition present called **spina bifida**. This means that the lower part of the neural tube (spinal column) does not close completely. These babies will have symptoms dependent upon the nature and severity of the birth defect.

Myelomeningocele, a form of spina bifida, occurs when there is a great deal of the nerves, muscles, and spinal fluid exposed—literally a hole in the lower back. There is a great risk of infection, and these openings must be closed immediately. These children commonly have problems with bowel and bladder control, as well as muscular control affecting the legs. A mild form of spina bifida is called **spina bifida occulta**, and causes no problems. In fact, this condition is usually found only when the child is being x-rayed for something else.

Approximately 1 child in 1,000 will develop a condition called **hydrocephalus**. Hydrocephalus occurs when there is more spinal fluid produced than the brain can absorb. This increased amount of fluid causes the child's head to swell. These children usually require neurosurgical intervention to create a shunt that will allow for drainage of the excess fluid.

What is cleft lip?

Cleft lip and/or cleft palate occurs in approximately 1 in 700 newborns. These babies can have defects in the palate (roof of the mouth) that extend to the lip, while others may have only a notch in the lip or a small defect in the palate. These conditions can usually be surgically repaired during the baby's first year.

What are some common genetic problems that may occur?

Down's Syndrome (Trisomy 21): Perhaps the most common and easily recognizable genetic disorder is Down's syndrome, which occurs because of the presence of an extra chromosome. In the United States, Down's syndrome occurs in 1 in 1,250 births—a decline from the 1 in 700 ten years ago. The reason for the decline is unknown. These children have physical features that are distinctive. These include flat back of the head, upward slanting eyes (mongolian features), small ears, wide spaced first and second toes; some have heart problems. Others will have large tongues. These children have an increased susceptibility to leukemia and infections. They are usually developmentally delayed. They may also have other complications related to the intestinal and heart systems. This disorder occurs with higher frequency in mothers over thirty-five years of age, or in very young mothers. Often, obstetricians will suggest that these mothers have amniocentesis, a test to determine if, in fact, the child will be born with Down's syndrome.

Cystic Fibrosis: Cystic fibrosis is a hereditary disorder that affects both the digestive and respiratory systems. Over 95 percent of the people who get cystic fibrosis are Caucasian, occurring at an estimated incidence of 1:3,100. Cystic fibrosis is prevalent in all races, occurring in 1 out of 14,000 in African Americans, and 1 in 11,500 of Hispanic births.

The gene for cystic fibrosis was identified in 1989. These children are recognized as having pancreatic insufficiency, recurrent respiratory infection, and increased salt in sweat. They will develop a chronic cough and have thicker than normal mucus in their airways. Additionally, they may have frequent pneumonia and large, foul-smelling stools. This condition is detected by your doctor when a "sweat test" is done.

The life span of these patients will depend on the ability of the family to prevent disease—i.e., good health maintenance. Life span has improved over the last few years, however the long term cure will probably lie in some type of gene therapy.

What sort of genital problems can occur?

Hypospadias is a condition where the urethral opening (called the meatus) is located on the shaft or underside of a boy's penis, instead of at the tip. It can occur anywhere on the penis, from the base to just under the glans. Surgical intervention is usually necessary and is usually done before the age of two.

My son's testicles don't look right. What is the problem?

Undescended testicles occur when the testicles don't descend into the scrotum. This may happen because of inappropriate response to the mother's hormones, or even a blockage that prevents their descent. Usually, the condition involves only one testes.

If both testes are not descended, there could be problems related to fertility, i.e., the child could be sterile (unable to father children on his own). Hormonal therapy is tried, initially; however, if the testicles have not descended by twelve to fifteen months and are not responsive to hormonal therapy, then surgical intervention is necessary.

My child has an extra finger! What will be done?

Extra digits on the hands and feet occur infrequently, but the condition is easily resolved. If these digits don't contain bone, they are simply tied off in the nursery. If the digit does contain bone or cartilage, then surgical intervention may be necessary.

What are heart murmurs?

Most heart murmurs heard in children from six months old and older are innocent. That is, they cause no real problems and go away as the child ages. In young infants, however, the presence of a heart murmur may cause your pediatrician some concern and require close evaluation and follow-up (see page 76). If there are additional symptoms such as cough, decreased appetite, and respiratory symptoms in the younger child, many pediatricians will request a second opinion from a pediatric cardiologist.

My baby has hiccups and sneezing—should I worry?

Most newborns have episodes of sneezing. It's simply their way of clearing the mucus out of the nasal passages—he is a "nose breather" initially. Hiccups are perfectly normal, though somewhat mysterious, spasmodic inhalations that will stop on their own and should not be a cause for alarm.

Medical Concerns/Problems in the First Year

What is asthma?

Asthma is a recurrent lung disorder characterized by hyperactive airways with swelling and blocking of the airways. Asthma can occur at any age but usually starts under the age of five. There is no single cause of asthma. It involves the immune system, the nervous system, infectious factors such as viruses and bacteria, as well as biochemical and psychological factors such as stress.

The lungs are essentially tubes that provide a pathway for the exchange of oxygen and carbon dioxide. These tubes are easily stimulated and very sensitive. When they become enlarged or inflamed, they may produce a lot of mucus and the tubes will become narrowed. As a result of this narrowing, you may hear a wheezing sound, especially on expiration (when your baby is blowing out carbon dioxide or exhaling).

What causes and "asthma attack" and how is it prevented?

Many things are known to trigger an asthma attack, including some known irritants such as cigarette smoke, infections, certain foods, and pollens such as molds and animal dander. The list is very long and your doctor will be able to provide you with more detailed information.

Once your baby's pediatrician has diagnosed your baby as having asthma, it's important that you monitor her breathing and know the right time to call your physician. You should call your doctor when:

◑ Your child's coughing and breathing have worsened—become more frequent or rapid

◑ Vomiting

◑ Your child is not responding to the medication your doctor has prescribed

In addition to medication you can do some "common sense" things to reduce the occurrence of asthma attacks:

◑ Try removing as many possible irritants as possible—pollen, cigarette, pipe, or cigar smoke, for example.

◑ Keep the house as clean and dust-free as possible.

What is bronchiolitis?

Bronchiolitis is an acute respiratory illness that occurs in infants and children under two. It is characterized by rapid breathing, wheezing, respiratory distress and chest retractions. Bronchiolitis is caused by viruses such as the respiratory syncytial virus (RSV), influenza types 1 and 3, para-influenza, rhinovirus, adenovirus, and occasionally mycolplasma pneumoniae. Respiratory syncytial virus accounts for the majority of cases in the first two years of life. The virus attacks the smaller tubes of the lungs and causes infection and inflammation. Wheezing occurs and many babies have significant changes in their ability to exchange oxygen and carbon dioxide. The younger the infant, the more severe the illness. Many are hospitalized. Bronchilitis occurs most commonly in the months between October and March.

Remember, bronchiolitis starts as a cold which progresses quickly to cough and wheezing. These babies may develop fever and become cyanotic (develop a bluish tint around the lips and fingertips).

This is an illness that you treat by treating the symptoms. I use salt water nose drops sparingly, or a humidifier, and I try to get as many fluids into the baby as possible. If your baby does not respond to standard treatment of fluids, humidification, and nose drops, call your doctor for advice.

What about the flu?

Each year, most of the United States is put under siege by the influenza virus, commonly known as the flu. This virus is classified as either A, B, or C, with various substrains. This means that each year we are attacked by a virus that is slightly different from the year before! If it is flu season where you live and your child has muscle soreness and pain, an acute onset of fever, chills, and a dry cough, you should contact your doctor for further instructions.

Most flu is treated with bed rest, lots of fluids, and acetaminophen or ibuprofen for fever.

Can my baby have pneumonia?

Little babies, just like adults can get pneumonia. These babies usually have difficulty breathing, coughing, and scattered wheezing. Most pneumonias are caused by a virus or follow a viral illness, and some can be bacterial in origin. Pneumonias, like most respiratory illnesses, are most often contracted from secretions and droplets (sneezing, saliva, etc.) from other children and adults. The children who get pneumonia are often in a weakened state from a prior illness.

You should suspect pneumonia or a significant respiratory problem if your infant or child has a cough, labored breathing, and fever, in addition to wheezing. Many times your doctor will confirm the diagnosis with a chest X-ray. If the pneumonia is viral, the care and treatment is symptomatic with fluids and antipyretics (medicine to reduce fever), such as acetaminophen and ibuprofen; if bacterial, fluids, antipyretics, and antibiotics. If the respiratory distress from the pneumonia is significant, your doctor may give oxygen to the baby.

My baby has either a hydrocele or an inguinal hernia—can you explain?

As your infant grows inside you, his testes grow in his abdomen. As time progresses, the testes move downward through a tubular area called the inguinal canal into the scrotum. As they move downward, the testes are accompanied by the lining of the wall of the abdomen called the peritoneum, which creates a sac that connects the testicle with the abdomen. Normally, the connection between the abdomen and the scrotal sac closes; however, in some boys, closure is incomplete, which allows fluid leakage into the scrotal area. This is called a hydrocele. If your baby has a hydrocele, your doctor will take a flashlight and shine it into the scrotum. It will light up!

A hydrocele will make the affected side of the scrotum very large. It is greater in size when the infant is upright because of the effect of gravity pulling everything, including leaking fluids, downward. Most hydroceles will resolve themselves by one year of age, as closure of the abdominal wall occurs. If it has not closed by one year, surgery is usually recommended.

In boys, an inguinal hernia occurs when intestine and accompanying peritoneum slip through the opening (the inguinal canal, described above) into the scrotal sac. Female infants may get hernias in the inguinal area when the peritoneum projection that comes down to the labia area does not close but remains open. It is recognized as a bulge in the area. Parents will tell their doctors about the "bump." Inguinal hernias in girls are uncommon. Your doctor will examine the area carefully, distinguishing the hernia from a hydrocele.

If you suspect a hernia, your doctor should be advised in order that he can evaluate it. Inguinal hernias will all eventually need to have surgery. This is to prevent the intestines from slipping into the area, becoming trapped. When this occurs, it is considered a medical emergency.

What is milk allergy?

True milk allergy is rare because infants are seldom fed cow's milk during the first year. The few infants who develop an intolerance to milk are usually those who are fed cow's milk in the early months. These infants will present to the pediatrician vomiting, diarrhea, and colic; others may be constipated. These infants may also have classic allergic reactions such as hives, difficulty in breathing, and generalized swelling. This is to be considered an emergency! Your doctor should be contacted immediately.

In those children who react to cow's milk, a milk substitute will be prescribed and milk products should be eliminated from the diet. If the reaction to milk is severe enough, medications may be used to treat the milk allergy symptoms. The key to treatment, however, is the close monitoring of feeding and elimination of milk products from the diet.

What causes vomiting?

Vomiting is regarded as the forceful projection of stomach contents through the mouth and/or nose, usually due to some type of infection. The spitting that occurs so frequently in the young infant after feeding is not considered vomiting. Overfeeding is probably the most common cause of vomiting in the young infant.

Pediatricians are concerned with vomiting in the very young infant, as too much can cause severe dehydration. The risk of dehydration, especially if combined with diarrhea, is very great. Of course, vomiting may be associated with or be a symptom of a more serious illness, such as sepsis (see page 84) or meningitis (see page 94).

Watch your infant to determine if anything is really wrong. One episode of vomiting is no reason to panic. Wait for at least an hour and follow with a small amount of breastmilk, formula, or electrolyte solution (do *NOT* give your baby cow's milk if he is allergic to dairy products or if he is under one year of age). Don't rush the feeding; just wait and see if the mixture is tolerated and increase the amount after about ten or fifteen minutes. Continue until a normal amount is tolerated. If you are breast-feeding, shorten the feeding time to test for vomiting. If none occurs, resume normal feeding.

However, if the following things occur, call your pediatrician:

◑ Vomiting persists

◑ Fever occurs—especially in the very young infant

◑ Signs of dehydration occur: sunken eyes, dry skin, no tears, doughy-feeling skin

◑ No wet diapers for several hours

◑ Sleeping too much

◑ The baby just doesn't look right!

What exactly is a cold?

The majority of colds—known as upper respiratory infections—are caused by viruses. As a rule of thumb, the average infant will get six to ten colds a year, lasting five to seven days! Most of the time, infants with colds have runny noses, congested breathing, and irritability.

The nasal passages of infants are narrow and swell easily. The drainage starts clear, and then becomes yellow to greenish in color. Colds are passed to your baby by droplets and secretions—coughs, kisses, and touching—from infected people. This is why we caution mothers to be careful about taking your baby out into the world when very young! If you must take your child out, choose carefully who touches him and remember that good hand-washing is essential for preventing the spread of the cold germ.

Most colds are benign and will go away on their own with little treatment. Watch for fever, suction the nose when needed, give plenty of fluids, use a vaporizer or humidifier, and lots of loving care.

How does one use a vaporizer or humidifier?

Humidifiers and vaporizers are used to add additional humidity to the air. It seems to help the baby breathe easier. When you use a humidifier you should:

◉   Make sure the unit is absolutely clean. Change the water daily; otherwise, you may set the stage for mold growth.

◉   Don't use anything except water in the unit. No medications should be added.

◉   Put the unit several feet from the infant's crib and allow the mist to circulate freely.

◉   Be prepared to change the baby's clothes, sheets, and blankets regularly!

Tell me about ear infections.

Ear infection—otitis media—is one of the most common medical problems that plague infants and children under three years old. It's the bacterial infection of the middle ear—the area behind the eardrum. Babies are more susceptible to ear infections because of the anatomical position of the eustachian tube. In babies, it occupies a horizontal position and does not allow for drainage from the middle ear as easily as in an adult or older child. When the tube is blocked and the fluid is trapped in the middle ear, the eardrum becomes swollen and discolored.

Ear infections are usually accompanied by fever, irritability, and ear pain. Small babies may rub the affected ear and you may see a discharge. This discharge usually indicates a perforation (hole) in the eardrum. If these symptoms occur, you should contact your pediatrician.

Tell me about "pink eye" or "red eye."

This condition is called conjunctivitis. The white part of the baby's eye becomes reddened, sometimes streaked. If this does not improve in a few days, you probably have infectious conjunctivitis. This condition can be caused by either bacteria or viruses. It is very contagious and you should institute rigid hand-washing, making sure the baby has his own washcloth and other toiletries. The child should not be taken to day care and the condition should be treated by your pediatrician.

If the white part of the baby's eye is reddish in the morning, but clears during the day, your baby probably has an allergic conjunctivitis, which may not require medication other than for itching. Many times, this clears by using warm towels to keep the eyes clear. If the discharge is cruddy and if the lids are swelling, it may be that the condition is caused by a bacteria or chlamydia. Your doctor needs to be notified in order for treatment to begin.

What can you tell me about tonsillitis and throat infections?

Babies under one year of age do get throat infections due to viral infection. No medication is necessary with a viral infection, but if the infection is caused by bacteria, such as streptococcus, medication is definitely called for. Complications from this infection include scarlet fever, and kidney and heart complications. Strep throats are diagnosed by using a screening test in the doctor's office. If the infection is not caused by streptococcus, your doctor will decide if therapy is required.

What exactly is HIV?

HIV, human immunodeficiency virus, is a chronic disease which affects virtually all parts of the body as a result of its impairment of the immune system. Currently, there is no cure for this ultimately fatal condition. Infants who have HIV have acquired it from infected mothers and usually develop the AIDS (acquired immunodeficiency syndrome) complex within a two-year period. There have been some promising therapies, but only time will tell how successful they will be.

If you have been diagnosed with HIV but your baby has not, be sure to continue to screen your baby for HIV at regular intervals. Current recommendations are that the child with two negative virologic tests, one of which is performed at one month of age or older, and one of which is performed at four months of age or older, is considered to be excluded from having HIV infection in the absence of clinical disease. These children, as a precaution, still should have a follow-up serologic test for confirmation of the absence HIV infection and seroreversion.

If your newborn has HIV, make sure the appropriate health providers are aware of the condition—especially your pediatrician. Part of the normal preventative care regimen for your baby, particularly immunizations, may need to be modified for your child. Your doctor should be aware when your infant develops colds and fever, or is exposed to any contagious disease, since the baby's depressed immune system will not allow the body to fight off infections as easily as with a normal immune system. Your pediatrician will discuss with you how to care for a child with HIV.

What is meningitis?

Meningitis occurs when the spinal fluid—fluid surrounding the brain and spinal cord—becomes infected. This is a very serious illness and constitutes a medical emergency. The symptoms can vary—fever, lethargy, poor appetite, tenting (bulging upward) of the fontanelles, stiff neck, vomiting, and irritability. Most often, mothers simply trust their instincts and say the child just isn't acting right! Watch your child closely and call your doctor immediately if these symptoms occur and go directly to the emergency room. The child will receive a complete evaluation, including a blood culture, and bladder and lumbar puncture to identify the organism causing the meningitis. If the doctors are convinced meningitis is a possibility, your infant will be placed on antibiotics and monitored very closely in the hospital.

Again, watch your child closely if these symptoms occur. The earlier treatment begins, the less likely complications will occur.

What are pinworms?

In the United States, this is a very common infection. It is a worldwide infection, estimated to occur in 30 percent of children. The pinworm has no respect for socioeconomic status. The main symptom is itching. The adult pinworm lives in the rectum and, at night, emerges and deposits eggs in the anal opening. As a result of the itching and scratching that occurs, the eggs are moved from fingers to mouth, swallowed, and renew their life cycle. Not a very pleasant picture, but very common!

You can make the diagnosis by looking at the worms on the skin of the anal opening. Your *doctor* can confirm the diagnosis by viewing the eggs captured on clear tape pressed against the anal area, then viewed under a microscope. The treatment is simple and consists of one or two doses of medicine; however, prevention is difficult as the worms have usually already spread throughout the household, requiring all members to be treated.

You can help prevent the spread by good hand-washing techniques—at home and by making sure the day care center is aware of the situation. Don't forget to wash your hands after playing with pets, too!

What is ringworm?

Ringworm is caused by a fungus. It is characterized by a circular patch on the head or body. Because these patches are circular with a smooth center, the name "ringworm" seems to fit. Ringworms on the body can be contracted from various sources, including dogs and cats. The scalp ringworm is usually passed from one *person* to another. Your child may have one or many lesions and will be treated with medications based on the severity and location of the ringworm. The length of treatment is also dependent on the severity of the illness, lasting from a few weeks to several months. Children with ringworm should not be sent to day care until the condition is under control.

What causes diarrhea?

Diarrhea is usually defined as frequent, watery stools. This occurs because the lining of the intestines is damaged, either from bacterial infections, viral and parasitic infections, food allergy, milk intolerance, or medications. It is considered dangerous, if prolonged, because of the threat of dehydration. Your pediatrician may try oral rehydration fluids and modify the diet over a few days with a bland diet.

What is impetigo?

This is a crusty, pustular rash that can occur anywhere on the body, but appears more commonly in the genital area and around the nose and mouth. It is very contagious and can spread anywhere there is an opening in the skin. Therefore, the use of separate washcloths is important and good hand-washing is essential. This problem usually occurs in the summer months and may surface after an insect bite or scratching and leaving the skin open. The same condition can occur during winter by rubbing a persistently runny nose. Your doctor will advise you on cleanliness and using an antibacterial soap and will tell you to keep the baby's nails clipped. He may also place your child on an antibiotic and topical ointment.

I've heard of roseola. What is this?

Roseola infantum is a contagious viral disease which develops quickly and is characterized by the rapid onset of fever in the 102–105 degree range. The fever usually lasts three to four days. The child will be a little slower than usual and seem a little sick, but not in proportion to the fever, which may seem raging to you! The fever will go away and a rash will appear on the face and upper body. This may last as long as one day and then disappear.

Temperature control is the only treatment your pediatrician is likely to prescribe. Keep the child away from other children until the rash is gone; except for the high temperature, this condition is relatively benign.

What are scabies?

Scabies is caused by a mite, a tiny bug that tunnels in the skin and lays its eggs. The rash that forms is a result of an allergic reaction to the scabies and its eggs and is very itchy. It's found almost anywhere on the body. The doctor may take a scraping of an affected area and look at it under a microscope to find the mite or eggs. If the diagnosis is confirmed, appropriate medication is prescribed. Sometimes, repeat treatments are necessary, as itching can last for several weeks.

My nine-month-old has very yellow-looking skin. Is this jaundice?

This is most likely due to a substance called carotenoids. They are commonly found in yellow vegetables such as carrots and squash. If your child ingests vegetables containing carotenoids in large quantities over an extended period of time, this phenomenon occurs. It causes no harm and does not need treatment. If you are very concerned, simply change the baby's diet and lessen the amount of carotenoid vegetables fed to your child.

What causes constipation?

Stool patterns are related to whether you are bottle or breast-feeding your baby. Feeding patterns, types of foods, family history, metabolic problems such as thyroid disease, intake, and the maturity of the baby may all contribute to constipation—i.e., a reduced number of stools, usually accompanied by incomplete evacuation. Also, some babies will have poor rectal muscle tone; or, the opening will be partially closed. Some babies will also have an absence of nerve cells in the lower end of the large intestine that makes stool passage difficult.

Premature and/or Low Birth Weight Babies

Unfortunately, for various reasons, babies sometimes come into the world before they're ready to be born, are born at less-than-ideal weight, or both. Though premature and low-weight births pose many serious health risks for these infants, there is treatment (which has improved drastically over the last ten years) and most recover to be perfectly normal babies.

What are the chances my baby will be born prematurely or have a low birth weight?

A mother's risk of having a premature child or a bad outcome to pregnancy will depend largely on her nutrition, medical and family history, lifestyle, environment, genetics, emotional stability, socioeconomic status, and medical care.

How small are these babies?

These infants are usually born before their full "term" of seven to nine months (the last trimester), and usually weigh less than five pounds.

Why are these babies born prematurely and/or so small?

Though it is extremely difficult to pinpoint the exact cause of a premature or low birth weight baby, the following risk factors appear to be major contributors:

Some Factors Contributing to Fetal Risk

Lifestyle	Physical environment
	Social environment
	Socioeconomic status
	Smoking
	Alcohol
	Drug Abuse
Genetic	Inherited traits
	Chromosomal problems
Maternal Health	Multiple pregnancies
	Age
	Weight
	Co-existing medical problems
	Emotional stability
	Placental implantation disorders
	Early membrane rupture
	Infection
	Abnormal pelvis size
	Intrauterine infections

How are these babies different when they're born?

Premature babies will, because of their small size and overall immature development, have sudden changes in their temperature mechanisms, becoming easily very cold or very warm. They will also have weak cries and may have trouble breathing. Some infants require either a respiratory machine to breathe, or additional oxygen.

How do they compare, physically, to the term infant?

When your doctor evaluates your baby, several different areas will determine her maturity. The areas most commonly judged are the ear cartilage, the creases of the foot, the breast-bud development, hair characteristics, and the genitals (see chapter 2). It is interesting that babies who are full term will have very "springable" ear cartilage in contrast to premature infants with "floppy" cartilage. As a rule, term infants will have coarser hair than pre-term infants, who will have thin or sparse hair. The skin on the term infant will feel smooth, while the pre-term infant will have very fragile, thin skin. Term infants will have palpable (something you can feel) breast-bud development in comparison to premature infants who will have little or no breast-bud development. In the term infant, you typically will find many foot creases; pre-term infants have smooth feet.

The genitalia, or genitals, of the term infant in the male will reveal large testes in a dark scrotum with many creases in comparison to the pre-term infant whose scrotum is usually smooth, and the testicles may or may not be felt. The female term infant will have prominent labia majora (outer lip) and clitoris, while the premature baby will have a prominent labia minora (inner lip of the vagina).

I've read that the premature baby's eyes may need special attention. Is this true?

Yes. Prematures need to be checked for retinopathy of prematurity. This disorder can occur especially if the baby has required oxygen over a period of time. All babies do not develop this condition, but it requires early detection to ensure successful treatment.

Premature infants are also at greater risk for developing eye disorders. These include strabismus (crossing of the eyes due to muscle imbalance), myopia (nearsightedness), hyperopia (farsightness), cataracts (lens opacity), and astigmatism (lens or cornea are irregularly shaped). In addition, the premature infant may develop other optic disorders.

How are premature babies cared for in the hospital?

These babies require immediate medical attention by a neo-natologist, a pediatrician specializing in the care of the sick new-born. The babies are kept in isolettes—incubators that allow control of their environment (temperature, humidity, oxygen, etc.) and protect them from the outside environment. When the baby's system has matured (when she is able to maintain her own tem-perature, breathe on her own, and requires little care inside the isolette) she will be moved into a regular baby crib.

Will I be able to hold my baby?

Depending on how the baby is progressing, you may be able to hold him for short periods of time outside the isolette. If not, you may hold and touch him through the special hand openings in the side of the isolette.

What about feeding the baby while she's in the isolette?

When mothers visit these babies, most neonatologists and pediatricians will encourage breast-feeding if the baby can come out of the isolette. If not, the mother is encouraged to express breast milk into a bottle for the baby to drink. Otherwise, the baby will be fed commercial formula. The important thing is that mom participate as much as possible in the care and recovery of her baby.

When can my baby go home?

Most premature babies will go home very near their actual due date if they are maintaining their body temperature, feeding well, and gaining weight. They may be behind, developmentally, for a couple of months or so, but with your attention and care, they'll soon catch up!

I'm nervous about taking her home. She's still so small!

Most parents are very anxious about taking any low birth weight babies home, but I assure you that your doctor would not release the baby if he were not absolutely certain that she was ready to go home with you!

One probable reason for your nervousness is the limited contact you've had with the baby while in the hospital. Another reason is simply that you've just been through such an ordeal. Some of you may even feel guilty—that somehow it was *your* fault the baby was born prematurely. But don't worry. All of these feelings are perfectly normal. It's time to get on with raising your baby! There will be some differences in the care of the baby initially, but remember that the doctor is always available to answer any questions.

What are some of the differences?

Usually, the baby's "listless" behavior is quite difficult to understand and can be frustrating when compared to the usually vigorous actions of the term baby. For instance, though the premature baby appears vigorous at feeding time, most of them will require significant amounts of energy for sucking—something they may not have because of their size and because their muscles are very weak. Most of these babies are bottle-fed and may require a special nipple designed to make sucking less of a problem. If you are breast-feeding, you may have to support her jaw as she's sucking.

However, remember that as the baby reaches his or her normal age action level, and as the baby's muscle and nerve coordination come together, activity will become more predictable. Until this point, it is important that we don't force these babies to do things beyond their capabilities.

This period in the premature baby's life can be a difficult time for young mothers and may require a considerable amount of additional education concerning the care of her baby and/or counseling from pediatricians and others.

Medical Concerns/Problems: Premature and/or Low Birth Weight Babies

What does "small for dates" mean?

The term "small for dates" refers to that group of infants who are born at a designated time but are smaller than expected at birth. Most of these infants are "term" infants (Forty weeks gestation) with premature size. They look like wise old men:

small, alert, and developmentally functioning at their designated age. Some premature infants can also be small for dates.

Small for dates infants usually are a result of the placenta not functioning properly, i.e., not providing enough nourishment for the fetus to grow. In general, these babies, after birth, will grow faster than usual with proper nutrition. Your doctor will also review the placenta and your history to see if there is a maternal reason for the small infant.

Is a premature and/or low birth weight infant given immunizations—and when?

It is recommended that the premature infant, if in the hospital and thriving, get the initial DTaP, hemophilus influenza type B (HIB), oral polio vaccine (OPV), and hepatitis B vaccine at the appropriate post-natal age.

Will my baby have any hearing problems?

Premature and/or low birth weight infants are at a higher risk for hearing problems. The AAP Committee on Infant Hearing in 1994 issued a recommendation that all newborns at risk for hearing loss be screened before three months of age. At-risk infants include those who suffered infections in utero (in the uterus), those under 3.3 pounds at birth, those who have bacterial meningitis, and the babies with APGAR scores of less than four at one minute, and less than six at five minutes (see chapter 2).

What about the baby's breathing?

Most episodes of premature apnea (irregular breathing including occasional periods of not breathing at all) appear to be related to the immature brain failing to send the signal for automatic breathing. The baby's heart rate will usually slow if he has apnea. Apnea can also occur because of infections and anemia. If your baby has had apnea, your doctor will treat him with medications which stimulate respiration. As your infant matures, the apnea and slow heart rate will improve. Your infant may be sent home on an "apnea monitor" to alert you if the baby is about to have a problem, or if one exists already.

What is respiratory distress syndrome?

This is a common problem with premature babies and is due to lung immaturity. In normal term infants, there is a substance on the surface of the lungs called surfactant that allows the lungs to have the elasticity needed to expand for breathing. In the last few years, neonatologists have been able, through treatment, to lessen the effects of this problem, or even prevent it through the use of medications given prior to birth or at birth.

Sometimes these infants will require the use of a ventilator for respiratory assistance. Oxygen is also given and is monitored carefully. Most babies improve over several days (or weeks) and require no further treatment, while others will require further monitoring and therapy.

What is an intracranial hemorrhage?

A premature infant, born at less than thirty-four weeks, runs a risk of bleeding in the brain. The more premature the infant, the greater the risk. The infants will usually have this problem during the first three days after birth. The approach to these babies depends on the severity of the hemorrhage. In mild hemorrhage, the doctors prefer to watch and wait. With the more severe hemorrhages, they will initiate vigorous and immediate treatment.

What about the baby's vision?

In prematures born in less than thirty-four weeks of gestation, there is a risk of retinopathy of prematurity (ROP). The retina of the eye develops and is complete in term infants. When a baby is born early, there is incomplete development of the retina. In babies who are at risk, the evaluation of the retina by a pediatric eye specialist is indicated after six weeks of age. Mild ROP will resolve with no treatment, while the more severe cases will require intervention.

Chapter 5

🪇

Feeding Your Baby

From Milk to Solids

Almost from the moment you first hold your baby in your arms, you'll realize that she is totally dependent upon you for the food and nourishment she'll need for the next several years! That's a daunting responsibility, but there *are* some answers to your questions! In this chapter, we'll talk about feeding your baby. Of course, with individual babies, it's often trial and error as to just what, where, how, when, and how much they will *want* or require in order to grow up well-fed and healthy.

The following questions and answers should give you some basic guidelines while learning and developing a feeding pattern for your child.

Please explain the five "building blocks" for good nutrition. What are they and what do they do?

The five building blocks are **proteins, carbohydrates, fats, vitamins, and minerals**. All are essential for a healthy body, but remember that too little *or* too much of *anything* will not bring the results we seek. Moderation and common sense play a big part in whether or not your child receives the right kinds of food!

Proteins are growth foods. They provide structure to every cell in the body and are responsible for growth, repair, and even replacement of tissue that is worn out or injured. Too little protein and the body will not function properly; too much and the body must work overtime to get rid of excess waste, expending energy better used for growth. Your baby will usually receive the proper amount of proteins in your breast milk, commercial formula, or cereal.

Carbohydrates: Carbohydrates are energy foods. Dietary carbohydrates include sugars such as glucose and fructose; disaccharides such as maltose, sucrose, and lactose; and complex carbohydrates, such as starches and dietary fibers. Disaccharides and starches are converted to glucose and absorbed in the intestine. They are also changed to glucose in the liver and used as an energy source for the body's tissues. Glucose is also converted and stored in the liver and skeletal muscles as glycogen.

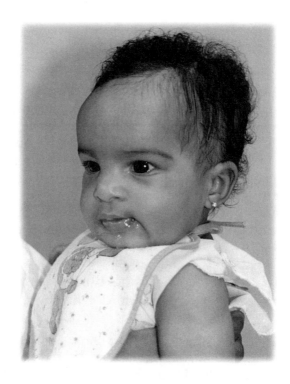

Good sources of energy from carbohydrates are found in breast milk (a primary source of lactose), dairy products, and fresh fruits and juices (which contain fructose and are quickly absorbed). As your child begins solid foods, appropriate amounts of starches (complex carbohydrates) can be found in beans, pasta, potatoes, whole grain, greens, etc. To avoid problems as your child ages, stay away from refined sugars—candy, icing, etc. They simply are not good for children!

Fats: Fats (lipids) are very essential to the body—especially in the young infant. Fats are important as a source for energy and essential fatty acids. Fats promote growth and babies need to grow. The key to fat ingestion is moderation. Cholesterol, a lipid, provides essential insulation for nerves in the brain and central nervous system. I do not recommend high or low cholesterol diets for infants. Mothers milk and commercial formula during the first year have the necessary amounts of fats and cholesterol for proper nutrition. Remember—moderation is the key word.

Vitamins: Vitamins themselves do not supply energy, but work with other foods to help the baby utilize his energy and grow healthy. The principle vitamins needed are A, C, D, E, K, thiamin, niacin, pantothenic acid, folacin, biotin, B12, and B6. Most term babies receive adequate vitamins from human milk, commercial formula, and food. Even if you have a picky eater, it is unlikely that he or she will suffer from a vitamin deficiency. Some vitamins are actually stored in body fat, so whatever the baby receives or does not receive during one day, the body will supply, though premature infants may require supplementation.

Minerals: Calcium, phosphorus, and magnesium are needed to help build bones. They are not needed in large amounts and it is rare to find a deficiency of these minerals in infants. However, there are two minerals that you should perhaps pay a little closer attention to: iron and sodium.

Iron is a mineral that babies need to help build hemoglobin—the substance in the red blood cells that carries oxygen throughout the body. Iron deficiency is not usually found before four to six months. Most babies will have adequate iron stores during this time. However, because of rapid growth, dietary iron is currently recommended to provide an appropriate rise in the total body hemoglobin. Iron supplementation is recommended at two months for premature infants and between four to six months in term infants. Breast-fed term infants are given iron drops and maintained on them for at least six months. Preterm infants on commercial formula are given iron supplementation as well as fortified cereal. For those children on formula, commercial infant formula and/or two servings a day of iron fortified infant cereal are recommended. Your doctor will calculate the dose of iron needed. You will usually be given only a one month supply because of the danger of overdose. During the first year—at around nine months—your doctor will do a simple finger stick (take a drop or two of blood from your baby's finger). He will then analyze the blood sample to determine if your baby's hemoglobin levels are within normal range. If not within an acceptable range, your child will be termed "anemic" (see page 83). One way to avoid this is to breast-feed your baby as long as possible. The iron in *your* milk is readily absorbed by your baby's body—more than with commercial formula or iron-fortified cereals. Also, avoid cow's milk during the first year of life. Cow's milk has very little iron and could irritate the baby's digestive system enough to cause small losses of iron over a period of time.

Sodium as sodium chloride (salt) is an ingredient we must watch carefully during the first year. Too much can bring about havoc on the body and cause fluid and water retention—too little can result in dehydration. Furthermore, although there is no evidence that the sodium content in the infant diet contributes to later hypertension, the myth lives on. You should be aware that since 1977, commercial infant foods have not contained any salt.

The best source of sodium for your infant is human breast milk. Commercial formula appears to contain an adequate source also, for the first year. A combination of breast milk or commercial formula and infant food allows for a low sodium chloride intake.

About solid foods—my grandmother says my baby could (and should) eat cereal at two weeks of age. What's wrong with this?

What's the rush? At two weeks, a child is definitely NOT ready for solid foods. I realize that a lot of this early feeding is part of a tradition, especially in the African American community. Mothers and grandmothers, through the years, have begun feeding solid foods at a very early age. ("That child is still hungry!" You want to starve that baby? Give him something to EAT!")

As a compromise, moms sometimes put "solid" food (which has been pureed or mixed with milk or other liquid) in a bottle with a bigger hole punched in the nipple. Commercially, there is even a plunger sold to feed solids! This mixture, fed to the child in this manner, can cause choking, but even worse, it is being fed to him before his delicate digestive system is ready for it!

The majority of babies between four to six months of age develop good muscle control of their bodies—especially the head and neck. They let you know they are interested in food by pushing their heads forward, and they are no longer pushing anything out of their mouths. From a developmental standpoint, their digestive system is maturing enough to handle solid foods.

Sometimes, you will only have to observe your baby's actions to decide that it's time for solids. She'll *watch* you eat, cry when finishing her formula as if she hasn't had enough, or begin to wake for feeding again during the night. She's trying to tell you it's time for something new!

So, although the advice given by Mama and Grandma is offered with love, try to hold off feeding your baby solids for a while. I assure you she's getting the nutrients she needs from her formula or your breast milk!

Breast-feeding

Speaking of breast milk—should I breast-feed my baby?

In my opinion, breast-feeding is the desired method of feeding your baby. Breast milk is natural, it's available all of the time, and it does not require time and preparation. Breast milk is also excellent nutritionally, and allows you to spend quality time with your baby. Mothers I've talked to report feeling relaxed when breast-feeding and that it aids in contractions of the uterus as it returns to normal size.

Not only does the breast-fed baby get excellent nourishment for its digestive system, but the child is naturally protected against some of the infections he may be exposed to during the early weeks after birth.

Obviously, human milk is the ideal milk for the human baby! It contains an appropriate amount of water to hydrate your baby, as well as calories and nutrients, such as minerals, vitamins, fats, proteins, and carbohydrates, which, though found in commercial formulas, cannot compare to the original!

How do I know if I CAN breast-feed?

Most mothers have the ability to breast-feed regardless of the breast size or nipple condition. When considering breast-feeding, you need to be aware of certain things which can make your decision easier: your attitude, prior preparation for breast-feeding, good nutrition on the part of the mother, and an adequate support system within the family.

Breast-feeding often depends on the flexibility of your schedule and can be very frustrating in the early days. I tell mothers to just ATTEMPT to feed according to the child's needs and that this will satisfy both of them. After several weeks working with a flexible schedule, the patterns of feeding usually stabilize and move from every two hours to every four hours.

When do I start breast-feeding?

I usually advise mothers to put the baby to the breast as soon as they feel up to it. Certainly, if they have taken any medication during the delivery process, they should wait until that medication has left their systems—usually this is within two or three hours. If they have not had medication, some mothers will begin breast-feeding right in the delivery room, which is perfectly all right.

However, the IDEAL place to begin is wherever you are most comfortable. Usually, that is in the relative privacy of your hospital room. (It is interesting to note that most hospitals in this country are not geared toward the natural breast-feeding method, but toward efficiency and convenience—in other words, the bottle!)

Who should know that I want to breast-feed my baby?

Make sure your pediatrician and the staff on the hospital floor are aware of your wishes and that they know you want the baby brought to you when he is hungry. Also, inform them that you do not wish your child to have a pacifier or a bottle.

My stomach hurts when I breast-feed. Why?

You will notice, initially, a cramping sensation in the lower abdomen, over the uterus, when you begin breast-feeding. This is called a letdown reflex and is perfectly normal and healthy and will subside quickly.

Will I be on a special diet?

Mothers who breast-feed should drink plenty of fluids—water, milk, juice—prior to feeding and frequently during the day. Other than this, simply eat a normal, healthy diet.

Will I need to give vitamins to my breast-feeding infant?

It must be stated that it is important for breast-fed babies that we supplement the breast milk with vitamins. Your doctor will tell you which type is best for you.

How should I hold my baby when I'm breast-feeding?

One of the most important things to consider when breast-feeding is that *you* are comfortable. Your position is important in making sure the baby is adequately fed. There are several positions:

When you are lying down, you should place the baby in an elevated position with the head resting on your upper arm in order to facilitate the movement of fluid in a downward direction. When you are in a sitting position, your baby should sit in the curvature of your arm and should be upright. Personally, I think that the relative safety of the sitting position is best for the baby. It allows you to see and observe your baby clearly during feeding time.

When your baby is sucking, make sure that his mouth has a good grip on the darkened area of the breast, the areola, as well as on the nipple. When the baby has a good grip, sometimes you may have to use your fingers to press the breast out of the way to be sure that the baby's nose is not blocked! The baby's sucking should be strong and steady in a smooth, rhythmic fashion. You can listen for and feel the baby's efforts and progress as he swallows the milk. Remember, good milk flow may take one to four days to develop.

How much should my baby eat at one time?

To begin, your baby will probably take no more than one to two ounces at a time. The amount will naturally increase as he grows and you will be able to tell, after some practice, when your baby has had enough to eat, or if he needs more. Some indications that he may not be getting enough milk are:

◐ Slow weight gain

◐ Diminished urine output

◐ Wrinkly or loose skin

◐ More crying than usual

Some signs that he may be getting *too much* to eat are:

◐ A lot of spitting up or vomiting right after feeding

◐ Abdominal pain—a tight, colicky reaction

◐ Excessive weight gain

How long should the baby feed?

I do not recommend nursing on one side more than five minutes at a time for each feeding during the first day or so, as your baby should be feeding several times a day. With time you can increase the feeding time to ten minutes—then fifteen minutes—several times a day. Usually, fifteen minutes on each side is enough so that most babies will be completely full. Remember to burp them frequently!

What's the best way to burp a baby?

Babies generally burp when they swallow air while feeding, either breast-feeding or bottle-feeding. If this air is not relieved from the baby's abdomen, he will swallow more air and become even more irritable. There are several ways/positions for burping. Perhaps one of these positions will be best for you and your baby:

When burping, place the baby in an upright position on your lap; place one hand over the chest with a slight pressure on the abdomen. Gently pat the infant's back, or rub in a circular motion.

You may also place the baby on your shoulder, supporting him with one hand while you pat or rub his back with the other.

My baby falls asleep while eating. What should I do?

Your baby may well fall asleep while eating. After all, he's full and contented in your arms ... what could be better than that? When this does occur, gently burp him to get him going again, but when he's obviously exhausted from feeding, stop until next time!

What about pacifiers between feedings? Should I use a pacifier at all?

This question has to be answered on an individual basis. If you are breast-feeding your baby, I suggest you do NOT let the baby suck on a pacifier. He should be put to the breast as often as possible—a pacifier between feedings could disturb the pattern you're trying to develop. After a few months and the baby has adjusted to the breast, pacifiers may be fine for babies who seem to need to suck on something, even when they are not hungry. The pacifier, for these babies, provides comfort and seems to pose no real problems. Whether or no to use the pacifier is a decision the parents and baby must make together.

What about breast-feeding twins?

If you have twins (and twins occur *most* often in African American families!) and intend to breast-feed, you will need to develop feeding patterns according to the demands of your babies. More than likely, they will be hungry at different times, so that feeding separately, and on different breasts, probably will be easier for you. However, by placing a U-shaped pillow beneath your twins for added support you may be able to breast-feed both babies at the same time, though you may find that the babies need supplementation from a bottle.

Is there anything special I should do to take care of my breasts?

When the baby has finished his feeding, it is important that you make sure your nipples are dry before covering them with a regular or special nursing bra. Also, experts recommend exposing nursing breasts to air for short periods of time.

Is it okay to use a bottle sometimes?

The use of a supplementary bottle is controversial. Many pediatricians feel that it is never necessary to supplement breast milk with a bottle; others feel that an occasional bottle is all right. I agree with the latter group. However, I do think that a bottle, especially during the first few weeks of the baby's life, should *not* be given. I say this because the baby needs to be able to suck on the breast regularly to establish a good flow of milk from the mother. The more he is put to the breast, the fewer problems you'll have getting the milk to come out! When supplemental bottles are given too often, the breast becomes sluggish from lack of use and it's harder to get the milk to flow—and therefore the baby to feed. Again, I'm referring to the first few weeks of life when establishing a pattern of feeding is important; after a couple of months, it's perfectly all right to supplement the breast-feeding with a bottle—either milk "expressed" into a bottle from the mother, or formula is used. If you do use formula, I recommend using the powdered variety—it has a long shelf-life and, in general, seems to be better tolerated by babies.

How and when should I begin to wean the baby from the breast?

Your baby should be nutritionally and developmentally ready for solid foods at about six months of age. My approach to weaning has been very flexible and consistent with the mother's practical and emotional needs. Usually, mothers decide when they are ready to wean the baby and then stop at that point. Some stop the breast-feeding at two to three months; others have waited as long as a year! When mothers indicate a desire to begin weaning their child, I have them substitute a daily breast-feeding with a cup or bottle and increase the number of cups or bottles as tolerated by the baby over the next few weeks. This procedure causes a gradual decline in the milk flow with minimal discomfort to Mom.

Are there any reasons NOT to breast-feed my baby?

Many of the reasons not to breast-feed a baby have to do with the perceived social stigma attached to the process, as well as very real physical concerns.

On an emotional level, there is often embarrassment, shame, and anxiety experienced in communities where breast-feeding is not commonly seen. After all, grown women are baring parts of their bodies not usually exposed in public! I have noticed mothers trying to hide the fact that they're breast-feeding—even right in the doctor's office! Another common response to breast-feeding has to do with the fathers. It has been called breast envy—fathers jealous that they cannot be part of this process that brings food and such comfort to their child!

Among the physical reasons for not breast-feeding are galactosemia, a condition where the child cannot tolerate lactose. Another reason is drug abuse, especially intravenous drug abuse, by the mother. These mothers usually have a high incidence of HIV and hepatitis which can be transmitted to the child. Tuberculosis (TB), herpes, or syphilis can also be transmitted to the child from breast milk.

What are some problems associated with breast-feeding?

The three most common problems are: 1) fatigue, 2) an anxious or uptight mother, and 3) a baby who is not sucking well.

Breast-feeding mothers MUST get adequate rest! You must learn to take advantage of the times when your baby is asleep, and rest when your baby is resting! Feeding goes better when you are calm and rested. Another problem may be engorgement. This is when the breast or areola becomes congested and full of milk, which can be very painful. The areola of the breast, especially, can become very sensitive because of the sensitive pain fibers in the area. The pain can be eased by gently manipulating the area or applying warm soaks to the area before feeding.

For breast engorgement, the first thing to do is make sure the breasts are properly supported. Cold packs should be used initially, followed by warm showers with soft rubbing of the breasts. Acetaminophen, if used in the proper dosage, should ease the discomfort and pose no problems for the breast-feeding infant.

The nipples of the breast (the areola is the area AROUND the nipple) can be another problem in breast-feeding. The most common reason for discomfort is the improper positioning of the baby's mouth on the nipple as he's sucking. His lower lip, positioned incorrectly, can cause the nipple to crack—the baby's thrusting tongue can cause pain on TOP of the nipple. Depending on how vigorously the baby sucks, improper positioning of the baby's mouth can be quite painful to the mother!

Your doctor can explain how sucking occurs and the proper technique for positioning your infant for feeding. Acetaminophen, if used in the proper dosage, should ease any discomfort and pose no problems for the breast-feeding infant. Also, when the nipples of the breast are cracked, make sure your breasts are dried properly after feeding. You may also use an ointment, such as lanolin or hydrocortisone, to soothe the area.

Bottle-feeding

Do most moms bottle-feed their babies?

There are any number of reasons why mothers choose bottle-feeding, some of which are: 1) some mothers simply prefer not to breast-feed their babies; 2) the mother's milk may be insufficient to satisfy the needs of their babies; and 3) sometimes mothers omit a breast-feeding, necessitating a supplemental bottle. An interesting note is that bottle-feeding seems to be on the upswing nationwide except in the western United States.

You must *not* breast-feed if you are taking any of the drugs listed below

Bromocriptine	Lithium
Cocaine	Marijuana
Cyclophosphamide	Methotrexate
Cyclosporine	Nicotine
Doxorubicin	PCP (phencyclidine)
Ergotamine	Phenindione
Heroin	

Check with your doctor to make sure any medicine you take contains none of these substances. The drugs of abuse should be avoided at all cost because of their effect on the mother as well as the infant.

Is there anything special I should know about bottle-feeding?

As with breast-feeding, there are general guidelines to follow:

(❶) Bottle-feeding is not to be rushed. Take your time and enjoy this time with your baby.

(❶) You should be careful not to overfeed your baby. As with breast milk, a few ounces should be enough to see how well she likes and tolerates the food. This amount will probably increase by one ounce per month until she reaches six to eight ounces. I usually do not recommend feeding, at any one sitting, more than eight ounces to an older infant. If your baby seems to have need for more than this amount, you should review this with your pediatrician. Therefore, initially, I recommend SMALL BOTTLES which hold a maximum of four ounces. As your baby's appetite increases, you can switch to the eight ounce bottles.

(I)   You should prop up the baby and NOT the bottle! Feeding is a process that should become a time of closeness between you and your child. Babies need the emotional and psychological feeling of security that comes from being held and talked to during their mealtimes.

(I)   It is important not to feel guilty about not being able, or about *wanting,* to breast-feed your baby. The important thing is that your baby receive adequate nutrition.

Do bottles have to be sterilized?

The question of sterilization is an interesting one. It is my opinion, and the opinion of many pediatricians, that it is not absolutely necessary to sterilize bottles if you have a healthy water supply where you live and if you use hot water with soap and a bottle brush to clean them. You may also put the bottles in an automatic dishwasher.

The nipples on the bottles should be washed and then rinsed several times. Run hot water through the nipples to see that the holes are open. If they are not, take a sterile diaper pin to reopen, or discard and use another one.

Notice that I said that sterilization was not ABSOLUTELY necessary. I do feel that, especially during the first few months, it is not a bad idea! Most communities have good, but not perfect water, and the environment of many babies may not be as clean as it should be for their safety.

How do you sterilize bottles?

There are a couple of ways to sterilize bottles:

The Aseptic Technique:

A sterilizer is used in which to place clean bottles, nipples, collars, and caps. You can buy a sterilizer, or you may use a large pot.

Water is added to the sterilizer/pot—enough to cover the bottles—and water is heated to boiling for approximately five minutes. The bottles and other related parts are taken out of the sterilizer and allowed to cool to room temperature before adding the formula and/or breast milk.

While the bottles are being sterilized, you will have another small pot in which you'll be sterilizing water for the formula. Mix the formula with this sterilized water and add to the sterilized bottles. Cap the bottles appropriately and refrigerate the full bottles. This formula may be stored for up to two days—just shake before using—and warm! (NOTE: I recommend NOT using a microwave for warming your child's bottles; there is a greater risk that the milk will not be heated evenly.)

Terminal Heating Method:

In this method, the formula is prepared according to the directions and put into bottles which have been washed. The bottles are capped loosely and put into a sterilizer. Water is brought up to about three inches, the sterilizer is covered, and heated to boiling for about twenty-five to thirty minutes. After cooling, the bottle caps are tightened and the bottles are placed in the refrigerator. With this method, the milk will be good for up to forty-eight hours.

What types of commercial milk formulas are available?

The two types are: ready-to-use, and ready-to-mix. Ready-to-use is formula that is pre-mixed with the necessary water and totals twenty calories per ounce. Simply pour it into a bottle, warm if necessary to room temperature, and feed the baby.

Ready-to-mix is concentrated in either liquid or powder. The liquid must be mixed with an equal amount of water (fifty/fifty). With the powdered ready-to-mix, there is a specified level of formula to mix with water to create the desired formula prescribed by your doctor.

In comparing cost, the ready-to-use seems to be slightly more expensive than ready-to-mix. As with most things, the "do it yourself" method always seems to save us money!

What about homemade formula?

I do not recommend homemade formula for a couple of reasons. In the past, many pediatricians recommended it because it was less expensive than powder or concentrate; today, however, there is relatively little cost difference. Additionally, it is very easy to mix the formula incorrectly, perhaps causing medical problems for the baby. Therefore, before you decide, I suggest that you check with your pediatrician for his or her recommendations.

How do I know which formula is right?

This will depend upon the recommendation of your pediatrician; however, before you buy the formula, be sure to check the expiration date stamped on the can or on the container. Also, make sure the can is not rusty or leaking. And it's always a good idea to read the directions on the container before using any formula. Different brands may have slightly different instructions for preparation.

Whichever I choose (bottle or breast), will my baby still need vitamins?

If you have taken care of yourself during pregnancy, followed your doctor's instructions, and are relatively healthy at delivery, your baby will not require any of the vitamin supplements if you are bottle-feeding.

If you are breast-feeding, Vitamin D (which is not present in breast milk) may be ordered by your doctor as a supplemental vitamin for your baby. You can also receive a sufficient amount of Vitamin D by simply taking your baby outside a few times each week! Vitamin D is made in the skin when it is exposed to the sun!

If, on the other hand, your baby is low birth weight or premature, he may require Vitamin D supplements as well as the other supplemental vitamins. Check with your pediatrician on this.

Your baby probably will *not* need additional iron for the first six months of life, as *your* iron stores and reserves protect her from anemia. After six months, however, she may need additional iron. This is, again, found in the iron-fortified cereals, as well as fruits and vegetables, but check with your doctor to determine which direction to take at this point.

How do I know how much milk to feed my infant?

This is a tough question, as needs of various babies differ. The normal guidelines are as follows:

Approximate Feedings for Infants and Frequency of Feedings under 1 Year

Age (month)	Ounces/Feeding	Number of Feedings
1	3–4	8
2	4–5	5–6
3	5–6	5

| 4 | 6–7 | 4–5 |
| 5–12 | 8 | 3–4 |

How do I get my baby off the bottle?

After approximately a year with the bottle, your baby will have become very attached to it! I suggest that, when you are ready to wean your child, you follow a similar weaning process as with the breast-fed babies. Substitute the bottle with a cup and appropriate meals while gradually removing the bottle. Remember weaning takes several weeks.

Remember *not* to let the baby sleep with the bottle at night or carry it around the house with him. These practices will not only make the child harder to wean, but as he's likely drinking more milk and juice, he may develop a poor appetite for other foods. In addition, your baby could develop "bottle mouth caries," or "nursing bottle caries," a condition which is a result of constant exposure of the teeth to sugar in the bottle, whether the bottle contains milk or juice. The longer the sugar in the food product stays in the mouth, the higher the chances the child will develop caries. Often, these children will sleep with a bottle or even carry them around all day in their mouths. They typically fail to eat properly and become anemic from lack of proper nutrition, and their teeth may become discolored and rotten. Additionally, carrying a bottle around takes away some natural instinct for socialization with other people! At any rate, by fifteen months of age, most babies have voluntarily discarded the bottle. There are so many more interesting things to pick up and carry around!

Solid Foods

Now that she's doing well with the bottle, I need to know about solid foods.

As with bottle- or breast-feeding, solid foods should be introduced in an atmosphere of comfort and pleasure and *never* rushed! You will adjust to her feeding patterns and she will adjust to the varied tastes and textures of this next step in growing up! She will also begin sleeping for longer periods of time and require less milk.

When do I start solid foods?

The question of when to begin has been debated for years. The current thinking, as stated before, is that the baby will be ready to be fed solid foods between four and six months of age. Just make sure, when you begin this next step, that the foods offered to your baby are valuable and will be utilized appropriately by her body. In other words, healthy foods! You should also remember that as you feed your baby, your attitude toward the feeding will have a direct impact on the baby. Attitudes about what *you* like and dislike could well affect what the baby personally accepts or rejects.

It is also important that the introduction of solid foods at approximately four months is only a *socially acceptable* measure, and not necessarily due to nutritional need.

What types of foods should I give my child?

Foods are usually grouped into five categories: 1) milk and milk products; 2) cereal; 3) fruits; 4) vegetables; and 5) meats. By nine months of age, I would expect that your baby will have had lots of experience with all these food groups!

How do I start feeding solids?

The first rule for feeding solids is to use a spoon—NO FEEDERS, NO BOTTLES! Human babies need to begin eating as older humans do—upright, comfortable, and with a spoon that fits their tiny mouths! And start with a very small amount of food—about a half teaspoon. Encourage him to eat and give him more if he seems to want it. He will have an easier time of it, too, if he is not too hungry when you begin feeding, and if you give him a small amount of milk before introducing him to the solid food. In other words, give him some milk, then a spoonful of solid food, then end with the milk. When he becomes used to the new solid food, he will require less and less milk.

How long should I feed my baby a particular food before moving on to the next food group? And which food should be given first?

I usually start the babies on rice cereal. It is a simple food—low in allergy reaction, easily digested, and absorbed well by the baby's delicate system. Mix the cereal with a small amount of milk (breast or commercial) and feed him small amounts as stated above. After your baby has tolerated the rice cereal for several days, you may try another type of cereal, but don't rush him! There is plenty of time and many different kinds of cereals. I recommend feeding your baby a single type of cereal for a few days (instead of several types) because this procedure will allow you to determine if a certain type of cereal causes an adverse reaction, such as a rash, diarrhea, constipation, or irritability. It will also give you a chance to learn which foods your baby particularly likes and dislikes.

What types of fruits are best?

Usually, at about six months of age, your baby is ready to begin fruits. I suggest you use the same pattern for feeding as with cereal—one type of fruit for several days, then another. You may also feed your baby cereal *and* fruit at this point. Remember that fresh fruits are always preferred to canned or frozen, but must always be pureed unless they are very soft to begin with. Your child will probably be able to digest apricots, pears, plums, bananas, and pureed apples or applesauce. Stay away from small chunks or pieces of fruit that may cause choking. Also, some fruits may cause the baby's stool to be soft or loose. If you notice this happening, be aware that you should not give this particular fruit too often.

What about vegetables?

Vegetables are often introduced after fruit, at about seven months. Again, use fresh or frozen, but all should be pureed for your baby in the beginning. A food processor or blender would be a good investment at this point.

The best vegetables for an infant's digestive system are squash, potatoes, carrots, and sweet potatoes, but try not to give any one of these in excess. Yellow vegetables may give your baby a yellowish tint due to the carotene in the vegetable. This is not a problem, but it has been mistaken for jaundice by new mothers! Of course, there will be some vegetables your baby will not like, but don't be discouraged. Feed him the ones he *does* like and make the experience as pleasing for him as possible!

Which meats are best?

Meats are usually introduced at around eight months of age and are traditionally the last solid food introduced. The best meats for digestion are lamb, beef, chicken, and pork. All should be very well pureed and well cooked. For home preparers, you should not add extra salt, pepper, or seasoning of any kind. Your baby will be chewing well by now and the digestive system will be performing at top capacity—a good thing, since he will likely be eating food in any or all of the food groups, plus drinking milk!

What if I don't want my child to have meat?

For those families who prefer going meatless, there are excellent balanced diets available for babies, which contain adequate protein sources. Nutrition experts have written several good books on the subject in response to the demand for vegetarian diets.

What if the baby won't eat what I try to feed her?

Occasionally, of course, you will introduce a food that your baby will not like. When this happens, try mixing the "good" with the "bad." For example, put a little fruit (something she likes) with the cereal (something she does *not* like) to see if she tolerates the mixture. This will probably work, but if it does not, try again with another combination! You will eventually find something she'll love. Don't be afraid to experiment!

The key to feeding is to take your time and allow the baby to do the same. Let her react to the food you offer. At this stage, she's just practicing, and if she refuses, it won't cause dietary deficiency! If she does not adjust after several days, then stop, try another type of food for a while, then start back with the original food. BUT KEEP TRYING! By the time your child is seven months old, you will have gone through most of the food groups and you will know which foods create problems.

If your baby develops diarrhea, wheezing, or rashes after eating certain foods, discontinue that particular food immediately, assuming that the baby is having some sort of allergic reaction. Make sure your pediatrician is made aware of this behavior.

Also, it is important that you learn to observe the signs your baby will give you that she's had ENOUGH! She'll close her mouth, purse her lips and turn her head away from the spoon, all indicating that she does not want to eat right now. DO NOT FORCE THE ISSUE! You want her to have a healthy attitude toward food and feeding. Being forced to eat when she's not ready will only make her dislike the whole process!

About how much food will he eat at first?

Initially, I recommend feeding the baby in small portions, i.e., one to two teaspoons at one feeding. A baby's stomach is *very* small (about the size of the *baby's* fist) and more than this amount could cause a lot of spitting up! The amount will naturally increase as he grows older.

What is "finger food" and when should she have it?

Finger food is just that—food that can be held in the baby's fingers. Most pediatricians, by the time the baby has reached seven months, will move to finger foods in order to prepare the baby for things to come. Your child may have teeth at this point, but if not, soft foods can still be "gummed" and swallowed by the baby in small lumps.

When starting with finger foods, make sure that the foods are soft and that the baby will not have any problems "chewing" or swallowing the food. Also, finger foods should be offered to your child only under your supervision!

Some good "gummable" foods you might offer your child are:

- ◑ Small chunks of soft cheese
- ◑ Macaroni and cheese
- ◑ Cooked and crumbled hamburger meat
- ◑ Stewed, soft chicken
- ◑ Whole-wheat pancakes
- ◑ Hard-boiled eggs
- ◑ Bananas
- ◑ Small pieces of steamed vegetables

Use your imagination and remember to make any of the "finger foods" soft, and HEALTHY!

While we're on the subject, I should take a moment to warn you of the other types of "small foods" that could mean serious trouble for your baby. It has been found that MORE BABIES DIE EACH YEAR FROM *CHOKING* THAN FROM POISONING. *DO NOT* give your young child these foods:

◑ Hot dogs

◑ Candy

◑ Grapes or nuts

◑ Raw carrot pieces

◑ Raw apple pieces

◑ Popcorn

◑ Lumps of peanut butter

◑ Cookies, biscuits, bread; *anything that does not dissolve easily in the baby's mouth!*

What about juices?

Most pediatricians will introduce juices during the second month of life—in diluted form. Others will wait until after solids are started and still others will wait until the baby is nine months or older. This group believes that you can avoid the acidic/eroding effect of juice around the teeth which can result in cavities. Also, most doctors will agree to delay the start of orange juice for the first year because of potential allergic responses.

Remember that even with formula or breast milk alone, you can provide adequate nutrition for the first year of life without starting him or her on juice. This is entirely up to you. My personal preference is to start your child on juice near the sixth month, feeding from a cup with a straw or nipple-type spout. This will also serve as an introductory cup.

When should the baby begin drinking from a cup?

By the time your child is nine months old, he will have developed enough coordination to begin holding and drinking from a cup. It won't take long, after you've held the cup to his lips a few times, for him to get the idea that maybe *he* can do *this* for himself! Of course, a significant amount will have been wasted on the floor and table before he becomes an expert at about ten or eleven months of age.

What kind of cup should it be?

One of the things I suggest is using a trainer cup that has a spout and is weighted on the bottom so that it does not flip over easily. Also, the two-handed cups seem to work .really well for young, not-too-well-coordinated hands!

When should I expect him to begin feeding himself?

Even before your baby uses the cup, he will be able to place food in his mouth with some sort of control. Of course, as with the liquid from the cup, there will be food all over your floor as he begins this new task!

What you have to keep in mind is that he is learning something very important, so giving praise for those chunks and lumps of food that actually go *into* his mouth should be *your* priority! Let him experiment as much as possible!

I suggest that parents use a very small spoon that will be appropriate for the baby's little mouth. You can find these small spoons almost anywhere—from department stores to the baby food section of your supermarket. I do not recommend using one of those plungers or feeding solid-type foods out of a bottle, i.e., blending milk and solid foods together and feeding from a bottle. I have seen instances of choking, aspiration, and pneumonia as a result of using these techniques.

Also, be careful that the baby does not overindulge by putting everything into his mouth at one time. Watch this very carefully! Just put some paper under the chair and enjoy this messy beginning to a newfound independence!

Commercial food seems to be so expensive. Can I prepare the baby's food at home?

Obviously, if you have time to prepare your food at home, do so. Home preparation cuts out a tremendous expense. In addition to that, you can control the seasoning as well as the artificial ingredients. Because of the increased interest in home preparation, there are several good books on the market (see the references section at the back of this book). Suffice it to say that if you prepare food at home, you'll need to invest in a strainer and a blender or food processor to prepare these foods.

A few guidelines for home preparation:

◑   Fruits, except for bananas, should be stewed. Apples, peaches, pears, and prunes should then be run through the food processor.

- Bananas should be very ripe and can be either mashed or pureed.

- I do not recommend the use of canned fruits consumed by adults because of the high sugar content.

- Vegetables, either fresh or frozen, should first be cooked, then put through the food processor. Squash, peas, carrots, and sweet potatoes are recommended.

- Some foods may come through your baby's intestinal tract in their original colors. For example, beef may be red; some green vegetables may cause green stools; squash and carrots or some yellow vegetables may also give the baby's skin a yellowish tinge if a large quantity is eaten.

- Meats should be well done before being pureed and very macerated in the food processor before feeding to the baby.

- I suggest to parents to always taste the food, especially homemade food, prior to feeding to make sure it is not spoiled or sour.

I don't have time to do this. Is commercial food okay?

Commercial foods are excellent alternatives for those parents who are uncomfortable or do not have the time needed for home preparation. The key to purchasing the commercial brands is to *read the labels!* All ingredients are listed according to their percentages; i.e., water may be listed first because the percentage of water contained in that particular food is higher than any other ingredient. As a rule, don't buy any food that has water as its major ingredient—except water!

Also, note the expiration date on the food container. As a rule, after opening food jars, cans, or bottles, do not keep either the milk or the food over two days (forty-eight hours), and never leave any opened food unrefrigerated.

What types of food should be avoided— and when?

Especially during the first several months of your baby's life, most pediatricians feel you should avoid, among other things, egg whites. This is because egg whites may cause allergic reactions. Peanut butter also has allergic tendencies and should not be given to a young child. Avoid giving your child any greasy, starchy foods, or foods with a high salt or seasoning content. (Review the section on the five building blocks to nutrition! See page 105)

Generally, I recommend that milk products such as cheese or yogurt NOT be given to your child until he or she is at least a year old.

Other foods to be avoided include fish, chocolate, cold drinks, sweets, and foods containing a lot of artificial ingredients. Hard candy should never be given to your child, not only because of the high sugar content, but because it's one of the things that can choke your child.

UNDER NO CIRCUMSTANCES SHOULD YOUR CHILD EAT "JUNK FOOD"!

No hamburgers, hot dogs, bologna, or other processed food-stuff. In fact, you should stay away from junk food for most of the formative period in the child's life. He or she will grow up healthier with good eating habits to carry him throughout his life.

My grandmother says that a fat or chubby baby is a healthy baby. Is this true?

Once upon a time, everyone thought that if your baby had little rolls of fat and dimpled knees and cheeks, he *must* be healthy! Now, as we've learned more about the body and about nutrition, we know that fat is not a sign of health.

Although it's not a certainty, fat babies have a definite *tendency* to become fat children; then, fat teenagers; and, finally, fat adults. This tendency has more to do with genetics than with what the child has on his plate. If his parents are on the heavy side, chances are, the child will be heavy also.

Fat or lean tendencies also have to do with the child's temperament—an active, "busy" baby will have a lower risk of obesity. A child that is very passive and easy going will have a higher risk. In other words, other than giving your child the benefit of a healthy diet and sensible eating patterns, there's little you can do about his or her physical tendencies! But take heart. Most chubby babies, by the time they begin to crawl and walk, will begin to loose that extra fat that Grandma thinks is so cute. And as long as they're *healthy*, you've done your job well!

Remember that the decision on how and what to feed your baby is often based on *your* personal history and how you react to new situations. Do you approach a new situation with a sense of adventure and learning? Or do you approach something different with fear and anxiety? Whichever type you are, please realize that the experience of eating is both physical *and* emotional—it's *everything* to your baby. *Make* it an adventure and a learning experience for him. You will be surprised and pleased when he approaches other complicated situations in his life in much the same way!

Your Baby's Teeth

Babies are usually born without teeth; however, some will occasionally get the jump on it and have a tooth or two when they enter the world! In many situations, the teeth may have to be removed. They are usually replaced later with the primary, or permanent teeth. But no matter when they appear, teeth are important and you need to know, right from the beginning, how to care for them!

Average Ages for Baby Teeth to Appear

Month	Tooth
6	Lower central incisor (Two bottom front teeth)
7	Lower lateral incisors (Two teeth on either side of the centrals)
8	Upper central incisors (Upper front teeth)
9	Upper lateral incisor (Upper front teeth next to the centrals)
10	Lower first molars (Big grinding teeth toward front side)
11	Upper first molar (Big grinding teeth toward front upper)
12	Lower cuspid
18	Upper cuspid
20	Lower second molar
24	Upper second molar

When do I start, and how do I clean my baby's first teeth?

A baby's first tooth usually appears at around six months of age. This is the time for you to begin prompt, *preventative* dental care of the teeth and gums. You should begin by wiping the teeth clean every day with a soft towel. As the baby gets used to your using the towel, and as more teeth come in, you may switch to a soft "baby size" toothbrush. Most pediatric dentists do not recommend the use of *toothpaste*, however, during the first year of life.

What happens when the baby starts teething?

As the teeth begin to push up through the gums, your child may well be uncomfortable. This is "teething." She may be irritable and begin to drool a lot more than usual. She may start biting down, hard, on your finger as you wipe her teeth. Many mothers, grandmothers, and pediatricians have also blamed teething for mushy stools, increased salivation, and low-grade fever, but, in the majority of babies, teething occurs without symptoms! You have to be careful not to mistake teething for a more serious disease.

What can I do to ease the pain of teething for my baby?

A firm, rubber teething ring that has been in the refrigerator may make her feel better. You may also try cool liquids and acetaminophen for babies. Patience and recognizing that teething is a normal phenomena in humans is important.

Does teething cause high fever and diarrhea?

Contrary to popular belief, teething in itself does not cause fever or diarrhea! If your child seems to be in real pain or has a temperature over 101 degrees, call your doctor. Her symptoms are probably caused by something other than teething.

What if the baby's teeth look dull in color?

The majority of babies will develop fine, white teeth. Some babies, however, will have teeth that look somewhat motley or are very soft. These teeth have a defect of the enamel covering, which, in general, will pose no problem, but should be seen by the dentist at the point when you notice that the rest of the teeth look the same way.

Can milk hurt my baby's teeth?

In terms of preventative care, it is very important that as the baby ages you should attempt to prevent as much decay as possible. There is a phenomenon called bottle mouth caries (nursing bottle caries) which results when the baby has been drinking milk out of a bottle over a long period of time. These babies are usually those who are seen with milk bottles in their mouths constantly and/or sleep with milk in their bottles throughout the night. The milk coats the back of the teeth and, because of the sugar in the milk, can result in tooth decay. You may also notice cavities in the first year from the same phenomenon when children are allowed to suck on *foods* with a high sugar content.

I prefer parents try to get the baby to sleep without the bottle at night, especially after three months of age. With babies who will not sleep without a bottle at night, use plain *water* or a pacifier.

I have always believed that, at a point when sucking diminishes, you will be able to throw the pacifier away with few problems.

What about fluoride?

The primary role of fluorides is to prevent dental decay. Fluoride, when it occurs in the water at an appropriate level, can lessen tooth decay by as much as 60 percent. If the amount of fluorides is below the therapeutic level, then it will be necessary to give your infant additional fluoride. Many communities in the United States have adequate fluoride levels in their drinking water, either as an additive or as a naturally occurring source. If not, your pediatrician will have to prescribe fluoride for your baby.

The American Dental Association's guidelines suggest that children living in an area with less than seven parts per million of fluoride be given supplemental fluoride from birth to thirteen years of age. Also, breast-fed babies may need more fluoride.

On the other hand, if too much fluoride is given, it may cause discoloration of the teeth. But don't worry too much! Just consult your physician about the fluoride content of the water where you live and he will advise as to the best way to take care of your baby's teeth.

Chapter 6

🐎

Living with Baby
Physical Concerns

Common Concerns

Occasionally, things come up concerning our children that are sudden and frightening to new parents. Always feel free to consult your pediatrician if a seemingly "abnormal" condition occurs with your child. Chances are, the situation will be temporary and easily explained and treated. Meanwhile, we'll discuss some of the most common physical concerns you may have to deal with.

What is a "normal" temperature?

"Normal" is a term that means different things to different people—especially when you are talking about babies. Your baby's temperature may go up and down about one degree during the course of the day. If you dress your infant in a lot of clothes in warm weather, her temperature may go up some; if she's underdressed in cold weather or cool climates, her temperature may go down. The normal ranges of temperature are: Rectal—97–100.4 degrees Fahrenheit (36.1–38 degrees Centigrade). If your baby has a rectal temp of 100.6 degrees Fahrenheit (38.2 degrees Centigrade) temperature, he would be considered to have a mild fever. If your young infant has a rectal temperature greater that 101 degrees Fahrenheit (38.4 Centigrade) you should notify your doctor, especially if your baby is less than three months old.

How do I take my baby's temperature?

It is virtually impossible to take an accurate oral temperature in an infant! They squirm, move their mouths, and may even try to suck on the thermometer. For a child less than twelve months of age, do a rectal temperature. Rectal temperatures are on average one degree higher than oral temperature. A 98.6 degree oral temperature would be 99.6 degrees rectally.

If your baby "feels warm," is irritable, or has some other illness such as a cold, you may want to take the temperature periodically.

The rectal thermometer has a nice short rounded end in comparison to the oral thermometer which has a long tapered end. Both are filled with mercury and both are fragile! When taking a rectal temperature:

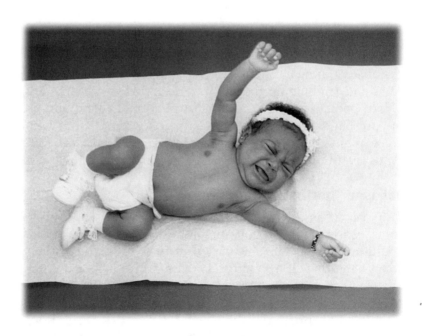

◐   Clean the thermometer by washing it in warm, soapy water, rinsing it, wiping it off with a wet towel or, if available, alcohol wipes or rubbing alcohol. After making sure it is clean, rub some petroleum jelly on it.

◐   Shake the thermometer until the mercury drops down toward the rounded end, below 96 degrees.

◐   Lay the infant over your lap, belly down, calm him down, then spread the buttocks open slightly and insert the rectal thermometer approximately three-quarters of an inch into the rectum. Hold the thermometer in place for three minutes.

◐   Read the temperature and write down the time of day and temperature.

◐   Wash the thermometer in warm soapy water, wipe off, and store in its container.

If you are nervous about using the rectal thermometer, you may use an axillary (under the arm) measurement. This is done as follows:

◐   Take the thermometer—either oral or rectal—and place under the armpit.

◐   Hold the infant's arm steady with the thermometer in place.

◐   Don't let the end of the thermometer stick out the other side of the armpit.

◐   Distract the infant.

◐   Keep in place at least four to five minutes.

Remember, the axillary temperature is one degree less than normal oral temperature. A fever in this case will be greater than 99.2 degrees F or 37.3 C. While axillary temperature measurements are easier, they don't appear to be as accurate, showing great differences (as much as three degrees) from the rectal temperatures.

In coming years, reading the temperature will be simplified by more widespread use of the digital thermometer. At present, cost and accuracy is still a problem.

What should I do if my baby has a fever?

◐   Make sure you take an accurate temperature (preferably taken rectally, but axillary is an alternative).

◐   Give the baby plenty of fluids.

◑ Dress your infant lightly—no heavy clothes.

◑ If the temperature is elevated, give a warm-water sponge bath for about twenty minutes. NO ALCOHOL RUBS OR ENEMAS.

◑ Monitor the temperature closely; if elevated, give acetaminophen according to your child's weight. Give NO aspirin unless specifically instructed to do so by your doctor.

◑ If your baby has a history of seizures, use warm-water baths regardless of the height of the baby's temperature. Consult your doctor if you have questions.

◑ If your baby is less than three months old and the temperature is greater that 100.6, call your doctor.

◑ If your baby's temperature exceeds 103 and the baby is just "acting sick," call your doctor.

◑ Consult your doctor if the temperature does not go down no matter what you do.

What is a febrile seizure?

Febrile seizures, or seizures with fever, occur in less than 5 percent of children between six months and four years of age. We attribute these seizures to a rapid rise or change in temperature. We do not think it is necessarily the level of temperature causing the fever.

If your infant has a fever and begins to have jerky movements or twitches, and does not respond to you, he is having a seizure. The seizures usually last less than five minutes (it may seem like a lifetime to you). Your infant will stop twitching or jerking after this period of time and cry or simply go to sleep. It is important that, if your infant is having a seizure, you don't try to stop it. Turn the infant to its side and call your doctor. He will probably tell you to go to the nearest emergency room for care. Drive carefully and do *not* panic!

Tell me about some allergies I may notice.

After about four months of age, you should be alert for allergies even though they may appear earlier. If the allergy appears to be related to something the child has eaten, you should immediately discontinue that particular food and inform your pediatrician of the symptoms you notice. Some examples of allergic reaction are:

◉ Skin rashes

◉ Vomiting shortly after eating

◉ Diarrhea within a few hours of eating

◉ Passing blood with the stools

◉ Wheezing

My child has some rashes and a birthmark. What causes this?

Birthmarks usually reflect an excess of one of the normal portions of skin in an area. Most common of these are pigment cells, epidermis, sebaceous glands, hair follicles, and blood vessels. Mongolian spots and salmon patches are the most common birthmarks.

Strawberry marks or salmon patches: Salmon patches, also called stork bites, are found in 70 percent of white infants and 60 percent of African American infants. These pink/red marks may be located anywhere, but are found on the nape of the neck in 40 percent of affected children. Some are found on the nose, eyelids, and the head. These marks usually disappear within the first month but can remain into adulthood. The neck lesions are the ones most likely to remain.

Mongolian spots: Almost 90 percent of African American infants have what are called Mongolian spots. These are dark areas usually present on the back or on the buttocks. Most of these spots will fade or disappear by the time the child is three years old.

Little blisters that peel off, leaving freckles, are called **pustular melanosis.** Usually these spots will disappear within the first month.

Milaria (heat rash): Sometimes you'll notice tiny, fluid-filled blisters, found most often on the face, neck, and chest, that are filled with a whitish fluid. This is called miliaria and is very common. Miliaria is due to sweat gland occlusion (blockage) or excessive sweating. If your infant is placed in a hot environment, this rash may appear. Conversely it disappears in a dry, cooler climate. It requires no treatment, just environmental sensitivity and lighter clothing.

Milia are tiny white bumps which classically appear on the nose, chin, and forehead. They are tiny cysts filled with skin proteins called keratin. They can occur in the mouth—usually at the top of the palate or on the gums—and are also called Epstein's pearls. Fifty percent of all newborns will have milia. No treatment is necessary. These disappear in the first three weeks of life.

Erythema Toxicum: The newborn rash, or erythema toxicum, is seen as a reddish area with white bumps in the center of the red splotches. It is seen most often shortly after birth, but rarely after a week. It may last a few hours to a few days and disappear. The cause of erythema toxicum is unknown and no treatment is necessary.

Hemangiomas: Hemangiomas are vascular in nature, meaning plenty of blood vessels. There are several different types and your pediatrician will discuss these with you if your child has one. Most hemangiomas have both a superficial and a deep part. They undergo a period of rapid growth, slow growth, and regression (start going away). This usually occurs over several years. As a general guideline and, depending on their location, most hemangiomas are left to regress on their own. If in a critical area such as the eye or mouth, or an area that can easily cause bleeding, surgery will be considered.

What can you tell me about jaundice?

Some babies will have a *yellowish* tinge to their skin and eyes which your pediatrician will call jaundice. Jaundice usually occurs within the first two or three days of life and is a result of too much bilirubin (pigment) present in the baby's bloodstream. This problem may be caused by the baby's liver being unable to break down and excrete (get rid of) the bilirubin. Jaundice can also be caused by an infection or blood incompatibility problems. These are uncommon, but if they occur, your doctor will inform you. Jaundice may last for several days until the infant is able to excrete the bilirubin. The majority of infants with neonatal jaundice do not sustain bilirubin levels of significance. Your doctor will monitor these levels carefully by using a blood test to measure the bilirubin. In those babies whose bilirubin is elevated, your doctor will use a "bilirubin light" to provide phototherapy, which effectively lowers the level. The infant is placed nude in his bed and the light is placed directly overhead and as close to the infant as possible. The light will be stopped when the bilirubin level is in a safe range. With managed care in many parts of the country, phototherapy is also being done at home in selected cases.

Breast milk jaundice is a condition that occurs in a significant number of babies who are breast-fed. They have bilirubin levels that are higher than normal. This is usually noticed sometime after the fourth day of life. This condition rarely causes a health problem.

If the jaundice occurs late, i.e., the first or second week of life, your doctor should be alerted immediately and the baby brought in for proper evaluation. Your pediatrician will then be able to give you further information on this condition and how it should be treated.

What sort of problems occur with urination and stools?

The newborn infant may urinate anywhere from fifteen to twenty times per day! Our concern is with babies who stay *dry* from four to six hours. These babies may be dehydrated or have other problems, such as an obstruction or blockage in the penis or bladder keeping the infant from voiding. This is usually a result of a congenital defect or abnormality. After the first few months, and during the first year, the baby may urinate six to eight times a day and may do so even more frequently, depending upon the fluid intake. If the urination is more excessive, you should notify your pediatrician to rule out any problems.

The baby's stools, initially, may be green/black, which may look alarming, but are perfectly normal. The green/black color occurs because a substance called meconium is inside the baby's intestines before he is born. Meconium is usually in the first stool passed. It is a good sign because you will know that the baby has no problems passing stools at this early stage! The stool color moves from a green/black to a greenish/yellow, from a mushy stool to a seedy-looking yellow stool, which is normal and is called a *transitional stool.* Finally, the stool will be a yellowish/brown and may be formed or semi-formed. Most babies who breast-feed will have softer, mushier stools than babies who are on commercial formulas.

For those of you interested, the average breast-fed baby has been known to pass up to twelve stools per day, versus the bottle-fed baby who will pass between four to eight stools per day!

How can I help my baby breathe easier when she has a cold?

When your baby has an upper respiratory infection (a cold with a runny nose) you may want to use a nose pump/syringe to ease her breathing if the discharge from her nose is very thick.

◑ Gather a medicine dropper, bulb syringe, normal saline, and small soft moist face towel.

◑ Lie the baby on her back on your lap or a flat surface where she is well controlled for movement.

◑ Place a few drops of normal saline in each nostril to thin the mucus.

◑ Squeeze the bulb syringe and then insert into the nostril carefully.

◑ Slowly release the bulb, thereby sucking excess fluid from her nostril.

What causes diaper rash?

When the skin is wet with urine, a change in the skin pH (acidity and alkalinity) will occur. When the baby has a bowel movement, there may also be a change in the pH balance which may cause a rash. Some babies will have more rashes than others and most doctors are at a loss as to why, except that some appear to be more susceptible to minimal amounts of ammonia in the urine.

How do I recognize and treat diaper rashes?

If your baby has an identifiable diaper dermatitis, your doctor will prescribe medication for the baby's bottom. The most common rashes are due to urine or stool coming in contact with the skin causing inflammation of the skin. At least 20 percent of all infants will develop a diaper rash. The basic types of diaper rashes that occur are the chafing rash, peri-anal rash, shallow ulceration type, and the secondary infected Candida albicans type rash.

How are diaper rashes treated?

Your doctor will treat all the rashes by asking you to make sure that the baby skin is kept as clean as possible from urine and stool. You must also keep the skin as dry as possible! I recommend frequent diaper changes and application of the necessary ointments suggested or prescribed by your doctor. The diaper must be changed frequently—especially at night. No rubber pants. I usually recommend exposing the genital area to air as much as possible. The appearance of the secondary infection— Candida will require prescription medications. Candida usually appears after a diaper rash has been present over four to five days.

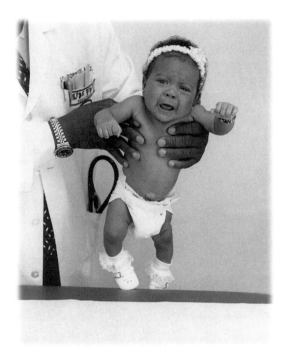

My baby has colic. Help!

Colic is a problem most of us are familiar with—either first-hand or by hearing stories from distraught parents!

We really don't fully understand colic. It is poorly defined. We do know that babies classically start with flushing of the face, drawing up the legs and crying at a high pitched level. These episodes are repetitive and may last for a few hours. The symptoms usually start several days to weeks after birth and are gone by the fourth month. It occurs equally in males and females. This paroxysmal crying is very disruptive in a family and can cause feelings of severe anxiety and guilt. Infant temperament appears to be related to colic. Those infants who are classified as difficult and those with a low sensory threshold appear to be at greater risk for developing colic.

Parents must understand that they must continue to offer comfort to their child and work toward realistic interaction with the child during this difficult time. Your pediatrician will take a complete history and do a comprehensive physical examination on the child to make sure there are no mechanical or physical causes for the colic. Your pediatrician will also explain the different factors that may contribute to the colic as well as its variable nature. Many methods of problem solving for the child and family will be suggested. Finally, remember that the usual symptoms will disappear by four months of age.

Fully one-fourth of the babies seen by pediatricians will experience colic at one time or another. In my practice, I have recommended relaxation techniques for parents, and suggested that both parents, especially mothers, reexamine their attitudes toward the baby. I also recommend time-tested basics such as frequent burping, warm baths, and wrapping in a blanket (swaddling).

On the whole, I have not been impressed with medications, but will occasionally prescribe something for colic as a last resort.

My baby spits up a lot. Is this a problem?

Many babies will spit up during infancy. In general this is not a major problem and may have to do with whatever position the baby is in. Some babies spit up in a lying-down position, some sitting, and others only when they're burped. The product will usually be curd-like milk and food products, as spitting up usually occurs shortly after eating.

Many of these babies simply eat too quickly and too much. The baby's stomach, after all, is *much* smaller than yours—as I've said before, about the size of a baby's fist. This should give you an idea of how much stretching and expanding has to take place as the infant eats.

Often the volume of milk spit out would seem to indicate that the baby is not really getting anything to eat! This is cause for panic with some new parents; however, as long as the baby is gaining weight there is usually no problem with spitting up. I am generally NOT concerned if:

◐   The spitting is drooling or dribbling;

◐   The spitting is milk-colored and not greenish; and,

◐   If the baby does not cough or gag during the spitting episode.

If YOU are concerned about this, there are some things you can do to minimize the spit-ups:

◐   Do not feed the baby when she is excited.

◐   Feed her in a quiet, calm environment.

◐   Make sure you burp the child gently and frequently.

◐   After feeding, place the baby in an upright (sitting) position.

For the most part, calm down, grab a diaper or towel for your lap and shoulder, and get ready! The spit-ups WILL happen!

How can I tell if the baby is just spitting up or if she's vomiting?

Vomiting is similar to spitting up and is usually not a problem unless it occurs frequently; however, projectile vomiting is another matter. In this situation, the vomit literally *shoots* out of the mouth.

Projectile vomiting is associated with pyloric stenosis, a condition which results from the pylorus muscle (located in the area from the stomach to the lower intestines) overdeveloping and not allowing milk to pass down into the stomach, thus causing milk or food to be forced back out of the baby's mouth. This is a condition that occurs infrequently and is found mostly in boys under two months of age. However, it IS a serious condition and your doctor should be alerted immediately, especially if this occurs several times during the day.

My grandmother told me about something called "thrush" and how to treat it. What exactly is this?

Thrush is a common medical problem that we have to deal with often. Thrush appears as white plaque that will not go away by wiping the mouth. It's caused by a fungus organism. Thrush can be found in the mouth and in the genital area.

In newborns, the organism that causes thrush frequently occurs when poorly sterilized nipple tops and pacifiers go into the baby's mouth. Home remedies for this condition don't work!

Your pediatrician will give you some idea of how to prevent thrush and will give you *medication* to treat it if it occurs.

What if my baby has diarrhea?

If your child's stools suddenly begin to occur with increasing frequency, change consistency, and change colors from light brown to greenish, this probably indicates a case of diarrhea. This can be a potentially serious situation and must be watched carefully, as babies, especially newborns, can become quickly dehydrated (when the body loses too much of its water). If you notice any of these symptoms, you should contact your doctor immediately.

Your doctor will want to know how often the child is stooling, the approximate amount, the consistency, the color, and whether or not blood was present in the stool. He will likely want to know what and how much the baby is eating, as one of his biggest concerns will be weight loss.

What do I look for in dehydration?

Dehydration is usually evident when the body loses excessive body water. It is indicated by several symptoms that you can familiarize yourself with. Dehydration may occur with vomiting alone or diarrhea. It most certainly can occur with both symptoms in an infant. Parents should, when their infant has vomiting or diarrhea or another related medical problem, watch for increased irritability or lethargy. Your infant will void less and there will be fewer tears. These symptoms accompany mild dehydration. In more severe dehydration, your baby can be irritable or increasingly lethargic, the eyes may appear sunken, the skin parched and not elastic-feeling; and voiding is infrequent. Your doctor should be notified, in either case, of these symptoms.

My baby is "grunting" and snorting a lot. What is causing this and what can I do?

If you notice a lot of snorting, snoring, or noisy breathing that seems to cause some difficulty for your baby, call your pediatrician. It may be he is having some trouble with either his tonsils or adenoids blocking the air passage in the back of the mouth.

No one really knows what causes the "grunting." You may think that your child is having trouble passing stools. This is not the case. Grunting occurs—the reason unclear—and usually stops by the fourth month of age. No treatment is required.

Lead Poisoning

I've been hearing a lot about lead poisoning lately. Exactly what is this?

Lead poisoning is a very common environmental child health problem in the United States. It's caused by having too much lead in the body. It can occur at any age, but is especially harmful to children six years old and younger.

What can lead poisoning do to my child?

Large amounts of lead in the child's bloodstream can result in brain damage, mental retardation, behavior problems, anemia, liver and kidney damage, hearing loss, hyperactivity, developmental delays, and various other physical and mental problems.

How many children are affected by lead poisoning?

In the United States, an estimated three to four *million* young children have lead poisoning; about one in six under the age of six years old.

How will I know if my child has lead poisoning?

An elevated blood lead level is the most positive sign of lead poisoning. Combined with symptoms such as irritability, sleep problems, abdominal pain, clumsiness, or behavioral changes indicate lead toxicity. A blood test is the only way to know for sure, as some of these problems may not be immediately apparent. It is recommended by the CDC (Centers for Disease Control) that all children be tested at twelve months of age. High risk children should be tested at six months.

Where does this lead come from?

There are multiple sources. The most common places are:

(I)   *House paint*—Seventy-five percent of the houses built before 1960 may contain old lead with concentrations of up to 50 percent lead by weight. Your baby could be poisoned by chewing on lead paint chips found on window sills; the lead "dust" gets on their hands and then into their mouths.

(I)   *Soil and lead-born emissions*—From car exhaust, smelters, incinerators, and from other industry waste products. This waste drifts downward, producing a high lead content in the soil. Children whose parents work in these industries are at great risk of exposure.

(I)   *Old playgrounds*—Decades of old peeling paint from playground equipment can drift down into the soil.

(I)   *Water*—EPA (Environmental Protection Agency) estimates that drinking water is the source of about 20 percent of America's lead exposure. This water flows through old lead pipes/service lines and lead plumbing. Even after lead pipes were banned, solder was legal for use on water drinking lines until 1980.

Other sources include imported ceramics and pottery, crystal and china, stained glass, and fish sinkers.

How do I avoid lead poisoning?

For the most part, just keep the baby clean; wash his hands and toys frequently, make sure he eats nutritional meals with plenty of iron and calcium, and keep the baby away from chipping paint if at all possible!

Chapter 7

🐴

Parenthood

Motherhood

As an expectant mother, you are experiencing certain growth stages separate and apart from any physical changes taking place within your body. The process begins as soon as you learn there's to be a new addition to your family.

I don't know anything about being pregnant or being a mother! How will I know what to do?

This is probably the first question you'll ask yourself—and anyone else you can find who's willing to listen. It's the first step in learning to become a mother. You've already had many valuable lessons from your own mother, but now it's time to begin thinking about your own ideas. Likely, you'll decide to do many of the things your mother did for you and your brothers and sisters, but you'll just as likely want to change a few things.

When you learn you're pregnant, you should start gathering information about babies and motherhood; from your own parents, friends, teachers, doctors, books, magazines—the sources are endless.

All this learning will help you to form a picture in your mind of just how it will be. But don't count on things going just the way you imagine they'll go. It's nice (and normal) to dream and look forward to your life with a new baby. Just remember that when the child is actually in your arms, you'll have to make some adjustments. That's the way it is with babies. The day-to-day business of mothering is rarely carried out exactly the way we planned.

I daydream a lot about what my baby will be like. I can almost *see* her. Is this healthy?

All mothers-to-be spend many pleasant hours daydreaming about whether or not their baby will be a boy or girl, dark or fair, quiet or rowdy, etc. These imaginings are quite normal and healthy and are an indication that you're investing some thought into your future relationship with your baby.

I have wonderful dreams about my baby, but I also have terrible thoughts sometimes. What if something goes wrong?

Try not to let your fears and any bad dreams upset you too much. It's also perfectly normal to experience some anxieties along with all the wonderful fantasies about your unborn child. Though these unpleasant wanderings may disturb you, they won't last and they may even have a positive effect by making you more aware of your responsibilities to your child.

I just brought my baby home. How can I remember all the stuff I've learned?

This is what I meant about things rarely going the way we planned! Your first days as a new mother will be filled with many conflicting emotions—much well-intentioned advice from almost everyone you come in contact with will probably just make things worse! It's virtually impossible to remember everything, so try to relax. Believe it or not, your instincts, coupled with the things you *have* learned, will serve both you and your baby quite well.

My friend seems to have no trouble at all with her new baby. What am *I* doing wrong?

First of all, rest assured that there is no such thing as a perfect mother. If you were to spend twenty-four hours with that friend who seems to have everything under control, I think you'd find that she, too, has plenty of doubts concerning her own abilities and that she often thinks that *you* are the perfect mom!

One of the best things you can do for yourself and your baby during this stage of learning is to *never* compare yourself to anyone else! You and your baby will work out your own ways of dealing with each other and both of you will be able to recognize whether or not your particular methods are working; i.e., you'll relax into a routine of caring for your child and he'll respond by smiling and enjoying the things you do for him. Always care for your baby in the way that *feels* right to you—even if it's not the way everybody else is doing it!

I think I'm finally learning something! But there's still so much I don't know!

That's the thing about children—we never stop learning about them. They seem to teach us something every day! What you're doing in this stage of mothering is getting into a rhythm—a pattern that will allow you to relax and experiment a little bit—thereby learning even more. And as you learn, your confidence in yourself will grow. Your friends and family will begin to notice and their praise will help you through those still-unsure moments. You may even be brave enough to offer some advice to that "perfect" friend!

I hear so much about spending "quality time" with a child. Who has time to do this after the daily routine of just making sure he's fed and clothed and sheltered?!

You don't have to ignore everything else in your life in order to spend quality time with your child! Chances are you're already doing it without even realizing that it's happening. Quality time is spent with your child as your changing his diaper and talking to him—watch him smile back at you! It's singing in his presence—look at him watching you with rapt attention; maybe even trying to "sing" with you. Tickle him as you walk by him during the course of the day—while you're doing other tasks—and watch him light up! Just knowing you are there and that you will be responsive to him is the best quality time there is.

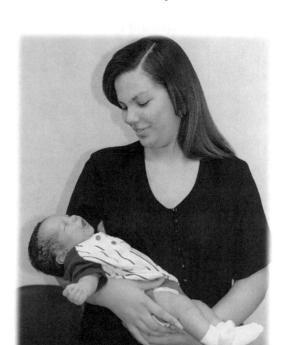

I'm really comfortable in caring for my baby. What could I have been so worried about?

Congratulations! You're finally in control. You've settled down and realized that to be less than perfect is just fine and that you're a pretty good mother after all. And you've discovered that, no matter what mistakes you make, your child *still* thinks you're wonderful! Of course, there are glitches in the best laid plans, but overall, NOT BAD, MOM!

Okay. I've done a good job, but *now* it seems that being a mother is *all* I'm good for! My partner doesn't seem to see me as a *woman* anymore—just the mother of his baby! What can I do?

As you take on the challenges of becoming a mother and finally get in the groove, it seems that your partner becomes increasingly confused about just *who* you are, right? Remember that it's probably very hard for him to associate "mother" with a sexual being in his life! And because you have so much to do, you're probably not doing a lot to help convince him that the flirtatious, sexy woman you were before the baby was born is *still* there—just subdued for the time being!

There are, however, some things you may try to let your partner know that you are still a woman, and still interested in him as a *man*!

◗ Obviously, being a fashion model first thing in the morning is virtually impossible with a baby in the house, but you *can* be at least refreshed when your partner comes home in the evening. If nothing else, wash your face and put on an outfit not spotted with creamed spinach! Brush your hair and smile. He'll notice your efforts, believe me! And *you'll* feel much better.

◗ Find ways to make your partner feel special. You've had a hard day, but try not to complain to him about it. Give him compliments and hug and kiss him when he least expects it. Let him know that he's appreciated and he'll return the favor!

◗ Make sure you include him in your activities and daily routine with the baby. If he has been gone all day, he's probably missed a lot. Share it with him; and ask his advice.

A Note for Single Moms:

Single moms, perhaps even more than moms with partners, may have a problem hanging on to the concept of "me." Many times we judge ourselves from feedback and through interaction with our significant others. Single moms living alone with their children are denied this, whether or not the decision to raise a child alone was by choice or necessity. Additionally, we sometimes see our own worth as human beings through the eyes of our family and friends. After a baby is born, it is difficult for family members (or almost anyone else) to see you as anything except a new mother! You may feel as if everyone has forgotten that you are still an intelligent, talented individual in your own right!

Often, if you're a single mom, the only direct support and feedback regarding your accomplishments comes from the infant in your arms crying to be fed! A screaming baby does little to convince you that you've accomplished anything worth talking about! You may even find it hard, at times, to *remember* how to talk to an adult! And what could you possibly have to say that would interest anyone? The most exciting thing you do all day is the laundry! Therefore, it is vitally important that you make every effort to surround yourself with caring, supportive people who understand what you're going through. Talk to family and friends, other single parents, community support groups. Seeking out these people and learning about *their* experiences as single parents can work wonders for your state of mind as you raise your child.

Your baby will benefit greatly from all the love and attention directed at him, but he'll *thrive* with a mom who is confident about her own identity. There is still a wonderful "grown-up" world out there, and you have a place in it! Give your baby your time and love, but save some for yourself!

I *do* ask my partner's advice about things; maybe too much. He seems to be better at this parenting thing than *I* am. Maybe I'm not such a good mother after all.

In the first place, you should feel privileged that you have a partner who is not only willing to help, but extremely *good* at it! Let him do his thing whenever he wants to! No two parents are alike, but both usually have certain things they're better at than the other. Recognize this and take advantage. Parenting, like marriage, is a partnership. Instead of venting jealousy, praise each other for a job well done! And remember, no matter what either of you says or does for your baby, when it comes right down to it, what do we hear? "I want my mommy!"

What is my role, as a mother, in the family structure?

You are already seen to be a strong, capable member of society and, because of this, a great deal is expected of you! But you will prove, against all odds, that you can deal with whatever comes your way—with grace and dignity.

Traditionally, Mama has been the one who's always been there; the one we turn to instinctively for love and guidance. It will be no different for your child. He will turn to *you* and you must be there for him, either as a single parent or one half of a couple whose primary goal is to instill in the child the *best* of themselves.

How is the father's role most often viewed within the family structure?

In past years, the role of the father was seen primarily as one of disciplinarian. Because of economic reasons, he was often forced to work several jobs to support his family. There has, unfortunately, been little significant change in this area. Today, both mothers and fathers have to work, necessitating changes in both attitude and behavior as more fathers share in the "baby rearing," and more mothers work outside the home.

Though you fathers may be reluctant, at first, to share in the "care and feeding" of baby, you'll probably find that by helping out, the atmosphere in the home becomes suddenly more relaxed! Mom has been relieved of some of the stress and guilt associated with leaving her child for work, and she will likely be surprised and pleased that Dad has decided to learn a couple of things about parental responsibility. Besides, this involvement will give you a head start with the initial bonding process, as well as establishing you as a vital part of the family unit early in the life of your infant.

What if the baby's father is not around?

Of course, the very *best* role model for your child is the baby's natural father, providing the father is stable and sincere in his efforts to participate in the parenting of his child. As I've stated, most men can *father* a child, but it takes an extraordinary human being to be Dad! In other words, if the baby's father is unstable or simply not there, use other male members in your family as role models. If there are no males in your family who seem willing to take on this responsibility, then turn to a good, consistent friend. Your child *needs* a strong male figure in his life to provide balance. There *are* dependable, strong, caring men out there. Find one!

I'm a single mom—divorced—and I'm not sure I can handle raising this baby alone. It's so much harder than I thought it would be!

Whether you have become a single parent through divorce or widowhood, or have chosen to raise your baby alone, you're apt to run into a few brick walls, and the emotional devastation brought about by any of these situations often leaves you ill-equipped to get over that wall.

Because our society, throughout history, has been biased in favor of two-parent families, support for those who have chosen or been forced into an alternate lifestyle is not the same as for the traditional family unit of mom, dad, and baby. Unfortunately, it's seen as an issue of either the "right" way or the "wrong" way!

One divorced mom told me, "The hardest thing—apart from never having enough money—is having no one to give me a break! No one to help with the everyday things. I'm with my baby—when I'm not working—*all the time*! I love him, but I don't know who *I* am anymore. I don't want to admit it, but sometimes I resent my child. And I guess he feels it, too."

I know how she feels. I want to be a good mother, but I can't do *everything!*

Most single moms have the feeling of being pulled in a hundred different directions at once, which results in a feeling of inadequacy—of not being able to do any one thing really well. These feelings, combined with the social stigma attached to single parenthood, can sometimes leave us feeling that we've failed as parents. However, I believe that as long as a single parent is making a sincere effort to raise a child in the best way they know how, *failing* is impossible!

The best advice I can offer is to make every effort to surround yourself with family and/or friends who accept the fact that you're a single parent and who understand your concerns.

There are thousands of single parents out there, just like you, going through the same financial and emotional upheavals characteristic of single parenthood. Seek them out. Talk to them. Share your feelings. Just realizing you're not *really* alone can make a big difference!

I'm sixteen. My boyfriend *wants* me to have a baby for him. I love him. Why shouldn't I do this?

First, let me ask *you* a question: What does *he* plan to do for *you* and the baby? As I've stated before, most any man can father a child, but it takes a very special, mature person to be a dad!

The same goes for a young woman who is considering becoming a mom.

The responsibilities (beyond conception) of raising a child in this day and age are ENORMOUS! *Most* men and women in your age group (though *you* may feel differently; may in fact *be* different) are not financially or emotionally ready for such a gigantic leap into adulthood!

Why take a chance on your young family becoming just another statistic? You've plenty of time to *really* prepare yourselves for being responsible, mature, loving parents—and your future children will thank you for waiting!

As a single parent, are there any particular actions I should take with respect to the absent parent?

One of the most positive things you can do for your child's emotional well-being is to NEVER speak or act in a negative manner about an absent parent! Remember that even an infant can sense anger and frustration. Try to avoid venting your frustrations about an absent mother or father in front of your child. Together or separate, you are both still his parents. Hostility and resentment from one or the other of you will only confuse and hurt him.

My baby's daddy is in the home, but seems to have no real "connection" to our baby. What can I do about this?

Many fathers seem to have some degree of difficulty showing affection to their children. The reality is that most are sensitive, caring men trying their best to overcome years of conditioning. The bottom line is that the man himself has to take the first step in breaking the stereotype. You cannot *make* him be a dad—he has to want to be one.

And since fathers and fathers-to-be are going through their own stages and may initially have different concerns, the next section of this book is all about fatherhood.

Fatherhood

You, as a mom-to-be, are naturally the one experiencing the wonderful fantasies and heart-stopping fears of the impending birth. Or are you? Just feeling your baby kick for the first time can convince you totally that absolutely no one could understand just what's happening to you—emotionally and physically. And you're probably right—to a degree. But besides your parents and other relatives, and your friends, there's someone else in your life who's most likely going through some big changes right along with you.

Your husband (or significant other; boyfriend, partner, etc.) is experiencing your pregnancy, too. He senses your vulnerability, mood swings, happiness and fears, and can see your body changing. This person is probably just as scared and confused (if not more so because he *can't* feel *exactly* what you're feeling) at the thought of becoming a father as you sometimes are at the realization that you will soon be a mother.

Like you, *they* too have concerns. The following questions have been asked by dads and dads-to-be. Feel free to share this section (or the whole book) with your partner.

I'm glad we're having a baby. I *think* I'm glad. But my partner is beginning to act differently toward me.

Try to remember that "different" doesn't have to mean "not good." Your partner is going through some dramatic emotional changes and is apt to take out some of her fears and frustrations on you. Also, her thoughts are quite naturally centered on the baby, especially during the first few months. She's concerned with getting ready—shopping for clothes and cribs, planning the baby's room, etc. Many men have little interest in these things yet feel left out when not directly involved. Conflicts often arise from this new experience. Try to be aware of both your feelings and hers, and keep the lines of communication open. Let her know how you're feeling. She probably is totally unaware of the amount of time and thought she's giving the baby and will be happy that you're willing to talk about it.

There's something else. She's not very interested in sex anymore.

Your partner is *not* rejecting you! There are an infinite number of things on her mind besides sex at this point, which doesn't mean she is losing interest in an intimate relationship with you. In fact, she may well need your closeness and support more than ever; just not physically—for a while. She may be tired, worried, sad, or nauseous—or all of these things, not to mention a little embarrassed at her rapidly changing body.

Many women cannot believe that their partners still find them attractive and still want to make love when their bodies are so misshapen. Show her that you think she's especially beautiful now. Intercourse, barring any complications during pregnancy, is possible right up until shortly before the baby is born, though you may have to get a little creative with positions! On the other hand, it may be that neither of you is particularly interested in physical sex, but don't let that stop you from being close. Just enjoying an intimate dinner or snuggling on the sofa can do wonders for the ego!

Again, talk with each other about this. Show her, as best you can, that you understand her feelings and that you'll be patient. Your relationship will soon be back to normal!

I'm willing to help out around the house, but everything I do seems to be done the *wrong* way!

Believe it or not, as much as they say they would appreciate a little help with a few things around the house, many women find it almost impossible to relinquish control of their households even for a moment! Therefore, during your discussions, your partner must make her wishes clear and there must be a definite understanding about who does what, and how. Both of you will probably need to do a little compromising—after all, your relationship is much more important than how the dishes are washed and dried or when the trash is taken out.

Men are supposed to be strong. She'll think I'm weak if I mention that I worry about things, too.

Keeping your worries and fears to yourself can only put a strain on your relationship with your partner. Remember that she needs your support and that, as your equal partner, she's there to support *you*. Talking about fears—birth defects, complications during labor and delivery, food, clothing, shelter, schools, doctors, time together after the baby comes, even fears of death for the mother and/or baby—all these things are common concerns for both moms and dads. Talk with each other about these things. Talk with other couples who've been through the childbirth process and survived! Learn as much as you can about the miracle of childbirth. Education, knowledge, and the sharing of what you feel are all keys to dispelling some of the anxieties.

What role can the father have during pregnancy?

I tell all fathers and fathers-to-be that whether or not the family operates in a classical setting with the man as "head" of the family, the mom and dad are "co-partners"; or if the father is not even a full-time inhabitant of the home, pregnancy involves *ALL* members of the household and requires tremendous psychological support from the male.

Problems arise when the fathers, lacking in both pride and consciousness, show little or no interest in the outcome of the pregnancy—or they simply disappear. A man participating in the *conception* of a child must realize that his participation has created a situation for which he should accept *equal responsibility with the mother*, and one which he should consider his number one priority.

Fatherhood should never be taken for granted. Most any male can "father" a child, but again, it takes a special person to be a dad. Fathers should be involved in as much of the pregnancy and pre-delivery room activities as possible. Attendance at Lamaze classes as well as birthing education classes is strongly encouraged. A cavalier or macho attitude does *not* work. You will discover that babies have a way of humbling the strongest among us, even *before* they're born!

My dad says men don't belong in the delivery room. Why should *I* be there?

The most important reason you should accompany your partner is simply for emotional support. This is a scary, confusing time and you can help her relax. The delivery room staff will likely put you to work—coaching her through contractions, talking gently to her, rubbing her back, etc.

Your dad was from the old school of thought that placed men in waiting rooms with boxes of cigars; men back then felt that the act of having a baby was the sole responsibility of the mother. These days, thankfully, we have learned a little more about sharing in the process of child rearing, not to mention participation in our children's lives from the moment they draw their first breath. I encourage fathers to be involved with the birth of the children from the very beginning. The father should be in the delivery room to watch the birth, not only for the psychological support, but to experience the thrill of the birth process itself. He should be with the mother and child as much as possible during the hospital stay and afterwards, at home. In short, he should be involved in every aspect of child rearing—from diapers to discipline!

Often, as a modern dad taking equal responsibility for the birth of your child, you'll be the first person to hold him in your arms. It's a special moment in the bonding process and one you'll treasure always. Don't miss it!

I try to help my partner, but I'm not very good at diapers and baths and all the other stuff ... all I seem to be able to do is play with him!

Though you may be all thumbs when it comes to diapers and such, you're helping more than you think, and the baby is not very particular about things at this point! And PLAY is absolutely essential for your child's emotional and intellectual development.

As a man, you're probably a bit more aggressive and vigorous, which will help your child develop physically. And calmer activities, such as reading to him or singing, will stimulate him emotionally and intellectually. Make no mistake, you are "playing" a vital role in your child's development.

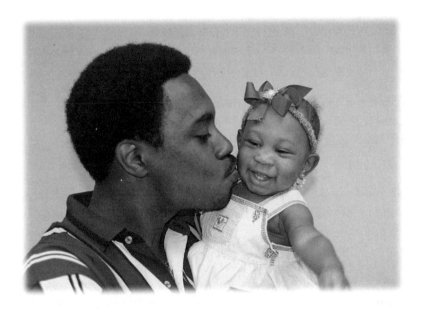

My partner spends so much time with the baby. She's always tired. What can I do for *her*?

The possibilities are endless! You could give her a break by getting up with the baby at night a little more often. Let her sleep late and then give her breakfast in bed while you take care of the baby. Take the baby with you for a drive or to a relatives' house for a morning or afternoon to give her time to herself. If finances allow, hire someone to come in to clean the house . . . use your imagination!

I thought babies were supposed to bring you closer together. It seems to be doing just the opposite to me and my partner. Why?

The most obvious reason is that you are both trying to cope with something neither of you were fully prepared for: the total dependency of and responsibility for a new human being; lack of time to spend together; new financial worries; and endless every-day tasks that were not required of you before the baby came.

That's why it's so important that the two of you sit down and discuss the "division of labor" in your new household, which will likely need to be adjusted from time to time as you and your child settle into the patterns of your lives. Remember that the more equal your responsibilities, the easier it will be to under-stand when one or the other of you begins to be dissatisfied with the way things are going. Communication of your feelings is es-sential for learning to share both the joys and burdens of raising a child!

I don't really feel like a father. In fact, I feel depressed about the whole thing. What's wrong with me?

It's perfectly normal not to feel like a father from the moment your child is born, and there's NOTHING wrong with you! It takes time to develop a relationship with this new little person, but make no mistake—you're this child's father for the rest of his life and your love and commitment to him, in whatever way you can show it, is essential to his growth and development! And you're his DAD. You're perfect just the way you are!

As for your depression, that's also a natural reaction to the extraordinary thing that's happened to your family. There are an infinite number of things contributing to the state of depression you find yourself trying to cope with: financial stresses, lack of sleep, a helpless (sometimes useless) feeling, a changing relationship with your partner, and a completely altered lifestyle!

For the most part, this depression will lighten up soon, as you and your partner adjust to your new baby and the changes brought about by her birth. Being *aware* of your feelings is the first step in being able to deal with them effectively. However, if these feelings persist, talk to someone in your family, your doctor, or a therapist. But try not to worry. The depression will more than likely go away as quickly as it appeared and you can begin to enjoy being a dad.

Babyhood

I've heard some things about babies' "temperament." Can you discuss this?

When we refer to the temperament of an infant, we are discussing how he behaves and the way he reacts to his environment. The characteristics of temperament were described in 1977 by Thomas and Chess and have remained the basis of most discussions of temperament. The characteristics are: ACTIVITY—motion during eating, sleeping, playing, etc.; ADAPTABILITY—ability or ease in adjusting or not adjusting to stimuli; APPROACH—how a child or infant initially responds to something new; RHYTHMICITY—how regular are functions of sleep, hunger, etc.; INTENSITY—how energetically a child responds to stimuli; MOOD—whether behavior is friendly or unfriendly in certain situations; SENSORY THRESHOLD—how much stimuli it takes to get responses; and DISTRACTIBILITY—how outside stimuli interfere. These various characteristics occur in clusters, creating some general categories: difficult child, easy child, and the slow-to-warm, or shy, child.

In our households, the way a baby "fits" is very significant.

Luckily, the "easy baby" category is the one seen most often—in about 40 percent of the population. Because of the lack of problems with these infants/children, and subsequent ease of parenting, and because they are so adaptable to various situations, we caution parents not to overdo or incorporate activities they may not want to remain as part of the child's normal behavior as he grows older. Also, because these children cause relatively little "trouble" within the household, we ask parents to be especially careful not to overlook them! If there are "difficult" or "shy" siblings in the home who require extra care, the "easy" child may be unintentionally ignored. This child, while a pleasure to have around, must nevertheless be taught how to discriminate and how to set rules for himself. Because he is generally very positive in his behavior, he may be too trusting with strangers. Make sure he knows the rules and that they are consistent with what he encounters in the outside world.

The children who have the complex of behaviors associated with the difficult child (about 10 percent of the population) have the hardest time adjusting to family life. These children do not adapt well to many situations and may be negative and unapproachable. Parenting these children takes a great deal of energy and persistence, but with repeated, gradual reinforcement for expected behavior, the child can learn what is expected of him and how to respond appropriately to situations in the family and outside the home. Patience with these children is vital.

The shy child (slow-to-warm) is somewhere between the easy child and the difficult child, accounting for about 15 percent of the population. These infants/children respond to a relaxed, patient atmosphere, and require a lot of repetition as they learn expected behaviors. Be firm, consistent, and loving without placing undue pressure on these children. Be a little flexible with a slow-to-warm child; not too rigid with the rules. He will respond to firmness, repetition, patience, and consistent reinforcement.

Whatever "type" your child turns out to be, a healthy, positive self-esteem in your child should be your ultimate goal as you practice appropriate parenting skills. Remember that the goals and expectations your have for your child should match his temperament.

To meet the daily challenges in the world today, children must be able to adapt to a myriad of different situations and people. It is up to you, as his parents, to interact with him on the most appropriate level. Remember, your baby is an individual! Your doctor should be able to help you understand and adjust to your child's behavior. If your doctor is unable to assist you, and the situation becomes too stressful, seek counseling with a reputable mental health professional in your area.

Why are role models so important for my child?

How many times have we heard, "You're just like your daddy!" Basically, that's a valid statement! Children tend to become what they *learn* to become. We all have many roles to play at different times in our lives. Your child will need to learn these roles and you, as his parents, will be his primary teachers.

Your baby, during this first all-important year, will learn skills and behavior patterns that will determine his intellectual and emotional maturity for the rest of his life. It's up to *you* to give him the best start possible!

I encourage all young parents to be aware that the image they project to their infant and child is one he or she will carry with them always. Your infant, though he may not be able to *tell* you, will "sense" trust, acceptance, and security from those around him. As he grows, his attitudes and behavior will reflect these feelings, whether positive or negative.

We all know (or remember) that small children, young, brutally *honest* children, will invariably embarrass us at the worst possible moments by copying and/or repeating everything they've seen and heard. And much to the chagrin of parents, they seem never to forget *anything*! (The preacher knows we have a little drink before dinner; our in-laws find out soon enough that we wish they'd *leave*; the department store Santa realizes, too late, that he has the worst breath in town ... well, you see what I mean!)

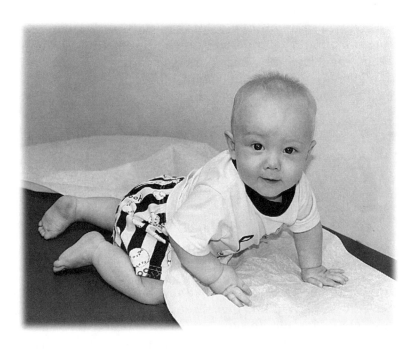

With these stories in mind, remember that your child's attitudes and responses to the environment and to other people will likely be very similar to yours, so make sure you stay on your toes and set a good example. A child is watching, listening, and *learning*, regardless of his age!

Adoption

Occasionally, for any number of medical, psychological, or economic reasons, we must consider alternatives to conventional methods of starting a family.

If you should need advice on alternate methods of starting a family (artificial insemination, surrogate motherhood, etc.) your doctor will be able to help you with the information you require; however, in this part of our manual, we will address the question of adoption.

I was told I cannot have children of my own. It is possible for a single person to adopt a child?

Increasingly, single parents are proving that it is not *absolutely* necessary to raise a child in a two-parent environment. Single persons, male and female, are showing a sense of responsibility and an awareness of the needs of children by considering adoption as an alternate method of starting a family.

There are, however, very serious matters to be taken into consideration when thinking about adopting a baby—single or married. I believe children available for adoption should be placed in the most stable environments possible. To that end, allow me to ask *you* a few questions.

◐　Why do you want a child?

◐　Are you serious about adoption?

◐　Are you prepared for the financial burden of not only the adoption process, but all the years to follow?

◐　Are you *really* ready to completely change your life? (And make no mistake, it WILL change—drastically!)

If you are not satisfied with your answers to these questions, maybe you need to think this through again. Remember, your decision will affect the lives of both the child and those close to him for a lifetime. I want that decision to have a *positive* outcome!

How does one start the adoption process?

There are no universal standards for adoption. Each state has its own rules and regulations, you should research the adoption process in your own state. There are various agencies that have children available for adoption and each agency considered should be checked out thoroughly. In addition, if you have secured an attorney, check him out—make sure he is reputable! Before adoption, make sure each step in the process is laid out in writing for you. You should make sure you have full disclosure of the medical information on the child and try to get any social or genetic history on the parents.

I've decided I really want to adopt. How could it go wrong?

In my experience, the usual causes of adoption failure are:

- *Unrealistic expectations:* Parents often bring a child home expecting the impossible—that everyone will immediately adjust to the new lifestyle a child demands. It simply doesn't work that way!

- *Financial problems:* A child is a big expense—for at least eighteen years—sometimes longer!

- *Mental or physical illness:* Sometimes, unfortunately and tragically, things happen to parents and children which are unexpected and/or unavoidable.

- *Inability to establish a relationship:* We have to face it—some people (whether adult or child) simply are not "made for each other."

I still want to adopt. What age child should I think about?

Most experts on adoption will tell you that it's best to adopt a child who's less than a year old. Somehow, it seems easier for both parents and child to develop a close relationship if it's begun early in the child's life. However, you'll find that most children available for adoption are much older. These children, more than likely, have been shuttled from one foster home to another and, as a result, are highly motivated and eager to begin new lives in a loving, stable environment. In other words, if you are serious about adoption, *all* children deserve your consideration, regardless of their ages!

Coping with Stress

It seems impossible that this tiny baby, this new life, could be bringing so much love and joy while, at the same time, throwing your once ordered, calm lives into complete chaos! The days, now, are like a runaway train and you're constantly rushing ahead to its next stop to prepare for its arrival. The unpredictability of its stops and starts, and your overwhelming exhaustion from trying to stay on schedule, could make a grown man cry—not to mention *you*—and the *baby*!

All this chaos—feeding, diapering, bathing, up at all hours, laundry—can be a cruel awakening to parents who've let themselves get lost in the *fantasy* that with a baby all their dreams of a perfect life will come true.

Now don't misunderstand me. Children *are* miracles; beautiful, fragile gifts that should be handled with care and reverence, but they are not always the perfectly behaved, always clean and happy little bundles we read about in books or see for a few seconds on television. The key to coping is to realize that you must find a way to *balance* the fantasy with the reality. When you wrap your freshly bathed baby in that soft, new blanket from Aunt Ruby, and she looks and smells like a little angel—understand that her *stomach* may not be aware of all your efforts. That new and improved formula you tried this morning may come up in a steaming mess all over the both of you—*and* the new blanket. Your awareness (and acceptance) of these inevitabilities can help you deal with the chaos and resulting stress of caring for your baby.

Okay. I can deal with that. But my partner just does what he's always done: in front of the TV, or out with his friends and not home at *all*. Why should *I* have to do everything?

As you've probably already learned, having a baby seems to change everything—and nothing. On the one hand, your life is not your own anymore. It seems you're an extension of your baby; not the other way around. That tiny little human has complete control over your every move! Everything is different for you and not at all what you expected, especially since, on the other hand, your partner carries on as if nothing extraordinary has happened. Right?

Unfortunately, the birth of a baby and the ensuing life changes they bring about can intensify any problems or difficulties already existing in a couples' relationship. The little things that irritated you about your partner *before* the baby can be blown out of all proportion *after* the birth.

His time in front of the TV can now seem to go on forever, especially when *you* can't find a minute just to go to the bathroom! And now, instead of enjoying some time to yourself when he goes out with friends, you feel angry and deserted just when you need him most.

To be fair, he *does* ask me to go out with him sometimes, but I have so much to do and I'm so tired. Then he gets angry. Why doesn't he understand?

Do *you* understand? How he may be feeling confused and rejected because you've said "no" to something you once enjoyed doing with him? And he probably doesn't understand that going out alone or with friends makes him appear selfish and insensitive in your eyes.

I guess that's the way we both feel. How can we change it?

Try finding time to sit down and talk about it. It's not going to be easy with all you *and* your partner have to do during your days. By the time you've finally gotten the baby to sleep, and your partner has dealt with hassles at work all day, neither of you may be in the best of moods to discuss the other's *feelings*. In other words, the discussion may escalate into an argument about just *who* deserves the most sympathy and understanding! If you feel it may turn out this way, agree to *postpone* your plans for discussion, but don't *cancel* them. It's important that you share your feelings and are able to come up with workable solutions.

My partner does help me, but now I'm going back to work, too. Shouldn't he do more?

This is something the two of you have to decide together. Often, even when moms return to the workforce, they still are seen as the parent most responsible for the household and for the care of the child. This can be an added burden and cause for more conflict and guilt—over leaving the baby in the first place and because she has even less time to provide her child with quality care. The husband or partner may also feel confused because schedule changes have necessitated changes in his own child-care responsibilities. Now, instead of simply coming home from work, he's sent to pick up the baby at day care; mom has to work late; the baby has diarrhea and there's only one diaper left; the grocery store has just closed; the car has a flat tire; and, it's just started raining.

I'm sure, on this day at least, your partner would feel he's gone way above and beyond the call of duty! Of course this sort of thing could happen to either of you. It happens to everybody at one time or another. We simply have to get through it. Thankfully, most days are *not* so hectic and for the most part go pretty much as planned. The point is that both of you work hard in different ways and you both must know exactly who's responsible for what and be prepared, as much as possible, for the unexpected.

How do we do that? Something unexpected *always* happens!

Write it down. Make a checklist for your family detailing just who does what. You can always switch tasks as schedules demand, or if agreed upon by the both of you. Knowing what's expected of you makes dealing with the *unexpected* a lot easier.

- Who pays the bills?
- Who cleans the house?
- Who takes care of the car?
- Who picks up the baby from the sitter or day care?
- Who gets up at night with the baby? (Try alternating nights.)
- Who mows the lawn?
- Who takes out the trash?
- Who washes and puts away the dishes?
- Who cooks?
- Who shops for food and baby supplies?
- Who takes the baby to the doctor for checkups?
- Who's turn is it to stay with the baby and give mom or dad some time to themselves?

What if I'm a single mom and have no one to share the chores with?

As I've stated before, being a parent is difficult, no matter what type of family is involved. Whether you are a single parent by choice, or because of a divorce or death, the stresses are much the same. If there is no one with whom you can share the daily chores of raising the baby, I would first advise that you learn to be very flexible concerning daily routines! Whether you are a working mom, or are able to stay at home with your child, the household chores will still need to be done—somehow! If finances allow, having a housekeeper at least once a week can help dramatically. Unfortunately, most of us cannot afford that luxury, and the dishes, laundry, and all the other chores just seem to pile up. This is the time when being flexible can pay off. Try to remember that the most important thing is the care of your baby. If the child still has clean clothes, put off the laundry for a day. If the baby has a cold and is irritable, leave the dishes until tomorrow. In other words, take care of the baby first; the house (the lawn, the trash, your dinner) can wait! Of course, there are obviously things we *have* to do, sooner or later, and being a single mom, you're the one who's most likely going to have to do them, but with a little advance planning and some flexibility, you can do it! Make your own list, relax, keep your sense of humor, and tackle the chores one at a time—when you *have* the time. If family or friends are not available to help you, just do the best you can. If you do your best, it's *always* good enough!

We've gotten the schedule worked out and it seems to be working, but we don't seem to be "close" like we were before. What's wrong?

Although it may be difficult, now, to see yourself as anything but the baby's parents (much less a partner or lover), you both need to make a special effort to remember how all this got started in the first place! You are still a *couple* and you have an investment in each other, apart from being parents. At some time during your busy days and nights, create moments when there's only the two of you. Sit down and talk about what you expect from each other and how you see your lives together as a family.

Arrange for a sitter and go to a movie or out to dinner—maybe just for a walk—but get out of the house and discover each other again!

Physical intimacy is something that time will take care of—after delivery and the first few exhausting weeks. However, being intimate encompasses more than sex. After all the both of you have been through, simply being close—holding hands, hugging, cuddling—can provide the warmth and caring you may have been missing and can reassure both of you that everything is going to be just fine.

All this is so confusing. We love our baby very much, but we never expected it to be so hard!

Please remember that you are not alone. I've never met a couple who weren't trying to cope with the same problems and concerns you're facing now.

Parenthood seems to bring out the best and the worst in all of us. One morning we wake and see an entirely different person sitting across the breakfast table and wonder where all that *attitude* came from! But instead of battling with it, try to think of it as a challenge; a normal reaction to an extraordinary situation that needs to be dealt with seriously and calmly. Usually, just talking with your partner openly and honestly will open lines of communication allowing you to *share* the anxieties and frustrations of parenthood, thereby lessening the tension between you.

Expressing Anger

A trait most recognizable in parents' anger and frustration toward their child is a tendency to feel that if the child is being impossible to live with, the child is doing it for a specific reason—on purpose—just to aggravate you. Just to see how much you can take; to see what you'll do; to make your life miserable.

It's easy to feel this way, especially if we *are*, in fact, feeling inadequate or that we're failures as parents. We somehow feel that the child *knows* this and is making every effort to be sure it's burned into our consciousness forever—to punish us or make us feel guilty for ever having had the temerity to believe we were capable of nurturing a new life!

The anger and stress seem to be in a dance—going around and around in a vicious circle; the child cries uncontrollably for hours; the parents feel frustrated and guilty at not being able to quiet the child; and the child (feeling their frustration and guilt) cries even more vigorously!

When we're angry, we're stressed out. When we feel stressed, we get angry, which *could* serve to relieve some of the stress; however, taking our anger out on those we love rarely relieves anything at all. In fact, we usually feel worse and even more frustrated and guilty.

Although these feelings are perfectly natural, human, and predictable (especially for new parents), we must try to recognize the factors contributing to this situation and try to eliminate—or at least *ease* them—before everything gets out of control. By this I mean that whether we explode in a rage or hold it all in and become withdrawn and depressed, our altered mental status can result in very traumatic episodes for our innocent babies!

Your *baby* will have absolutely no idea what brought about your outburst. He will only be startled or frightened. As far as the bottling-up of your feelings, the baby will feel only the absence and loss of your smiling face and laughing voice. Either way, he'll suffer without the slightest idea of how this disturbing thing could have happened! Furthermore, if you, as an extension of your anger, lash out at him with physical force or some sort of rough treatment or yelling, he will be totally amazed, confused, and scared. Try to understand that he knows *nothing* of your troubles or your anger. It is not his concern at this young age!

All of us get angry. All of us feel stress. What we have to do is try to remember that our infants cannot be blamed for *our* anger, and any punishment for expressing his needs in the only way he knows how—by crying—has no effect at all. He simply does not understand.

As much as possible, we must try to see the humor in our daily lives—to realize that the situation creating our tension will get better; it's *not*, in all probability, as bad as it seems; and, it is NOT THE BABY'S FAULT!

So, instead of hitting, shaking, or yelling at a child who only wants to love you, step back, take a deep breath, and hug your child instead. You'll be surprised how much his sweet response can relieve that anger and stress! His love is unconditional. Yours should be, too!

I really get angry sometimes. What can I do to relieve it?

Some things that may work for you are:

◑   Try to determine EXACTLY what it is that has made you angry in the first place. (Is it *really* the baby's crying and spitting up all day that has you on edge, or is it because your partner has not been home to help out?)

◑   Find a few moments to sit by yourself and take some deep breaths until you calm down. Throwing a tantrum and screaming at your family rarely solves anything; usually things get worse!

◑   Now that you've determined *what* has made you angry, make an effort to *explain*, as clearly as possible, the reason you're upset, and why (even if it's only your infant at home to listen to you, it always helps to get it off your chest!) and instead of yelling, speak in a slow, quiet voice.

◑   Last, but certainly not least, keep a sense of humor about the everyday trials and pressures that come with raising a baby. We forget sometimes that we're only human. None of us are perfect and never will be! Find the humor in your imperfections and in difficult situations and take a break from anger!

Substance Abuse

We live in a society where the use of drugs, including alcohol, is widespread and in many cases permissible. Substance abuse crosses gender, ethnic, cultural, geographic, and socioeconomic lines. Alcoholism and the dependence on psychoactive substances are forms of chemical dependency—the physical and psychological reliance on a chemical. Substance abuse has no simple etiology. Factors which contribute range from genetic predisposition to behaviors such as delinquency, poor self-control, anxiety, and low self-esteem. Family attitudes and stresses as well as social pressures contribute to the problem.

The effects of substance abuse are frequently seen with "people getting high": change in attitude and violation of rules and values, overdoses, loss of control, paranoid behavior, physical degeneration, bizarre sleep and eating habits, and suicidal gestures. There is a need to abuse daily in order to feel "normal."

With education and abstinence, most of the problems related to substance abuse and their effect on the infant would be prevented.

What drugs are most commonly abused in this country?

The drugs most commonly abused are: marijuana, heroin, cocaine, and alcohol.

How is cocaine used, and what is its effect on the newborn?

Cocaine is commonly used by inhaling (snorting) the powder through the nose or smoking as crack. It can be inhaled (free-based) or injected intravenously. It is used in combination with alcohol, sedatives, marijuana, hypnotics (especially downers), and cigarettes. It is cheap. It is short lived—having a half-life of ten minutes. This leads to frequent use and subsequent addiction.

Pregnant women who use cocaine are more likely to lose their babies or experience the pain of having their infant born dead. The babies who live are frequently smaller in weight and length and have smaller heads. These babies may have problems even before birth, which are usually related to the poor nutritional health care of the mothers—i.e., many of these mothers receive little or no health care guidance during pregnancy. Babies born to addicted mothers commonly have a higher incidence of infectious diseases, and can have sexually transmitted diseases passed on to them from an infected mother. PREVENTION: DON'T USE COCAINE DURING PREGNANCY (or at any time).

What is the effect of heroin usage?

Heroin is a drug that crosses the placenta easily. It virtually saturates the fetal tissues in mothers who are heroin addicted. At least half of these infants are low birth weight and half are small for dates. There is a higher number of still births (babies born dead) in addicted mothers. Within forty-eight hours of birth the majority of these infants have withdrawal symptoms. The severity of the withdrawal is associated with the severity of addiction in the mother, the timing of her last dose, and the strength of her dosage. Infants of addicted mothers in withdrawal are very irritable, may have vomiting or diarrhea, poor temperature control, and seizures. Many of these infants will require other drugs to ease the symptoms. Withdrawal can take as long as several weeks. Currently, information is being gathered around the country; however, experience has shown that these infants have many problems. Many are placed in foster care. Most have poor access to health care services. In school, many have problems with aggressiveness and have attention and concentration problems. Prevention: NO HEROIN DURING PREGNANCY (or at any time).

How does marijuana affect the newborn?

Marijuana is another drug that is abused during pregnancy; in many cases the pregnancy does not go to full term. These babies are usually smaller in weight and height, though the head appears to be normal.

Though it's harmful to an unborn child, the mothers appear to be more affected by the use of marijuana than are their babies. It is *after* the birth, with the mothers continued use of the drug, that the babies may suffer; i.e., through neglect and possibly abuse because of the effect of the mother's dependency on the drug.

How does alcohol affect the fetus?

Alcohol causes a distinct syndrome in the unborn infant which is called fetal alcohol syndrome. It is believed to occur as often as 1 in every 1,000 live births to infants of mothers who drink alcohol during pregnancy. Fetal alcohol syndrome usually causes the baby to have a small head, flattened nose, and an unusual-looking upper lip. There may be some poor development of the fingernails and toenails, and sometimes the baby will have a heart defect. Many of these infants will be mentally retarded. Others will develop short attention spans, high activity levels, and learning problems. They may develop hearing loss. FAS is a totally preventable problem. With appropriate education on the hazards of drinking during pregnancy, FAS would not exist.

It is not known, at this point in time, just how much alcohol causes this syndrome. To be safe: NO DRINKING DURING PREGNANCY!

Child Abuse

All of us know something about abuse—hopefully our knowledge is not firsthand—but most of us are helpless to explain it. We can only speculate that it is somehow related to stress and socio-economic conditions.

Unfortunately, child (and baby) abuse appears to be on the rise. Perhaps simply because of the advances in media technology, we are able to hear about it and see it more readily now than in the past.

At any rate, the instances of abuse are staggering. It is estimated that over 500,000 children are abused yearly. Many feel that the additional stresses and strains that affect Americans in general have a definite bearing on this increase. In the African American community, for example, two out of three infants live in a female-headed household, often in poverty. The medium income of black parents is significantly lower than that of whites, and the worry about the basics, such as food, clothing, and shelter, are often completely debilitating. Anger over this situation, sometimes born out of frustration, but most of the time from unknown factors, may lead to abuse. It certainly leads to stress. But remember: ABUSE IS NOT NECESSARILY THE *PHYSICAL* BEATING OF AN INFANT.

What are the types of abuse?

There are many different types of abuse, which may fall into one of the following four categories:

Physical Abuse: If a child is being physically abused, he will more than likely have visible signs, such as bruises, burns, cuts, abrasions, broken bones, etc. He may have been shaken, beaten, burned—all by someone he knows or as a victim of random violence.

Emotional Abuse: Emotional or mental abuse most often manifests itself in the form of verbal abuse, used to either belittle or terrorize a child. How many times have you seen a parent in the supermarket or department store not only slap or hit a child, but yell ugly, threatening words because the child was perceived as misbehaving? One can only guess at what the child is forced to endure in the privacy of his own home.

Sexual Abuse: Sexual abuse refers to the contact or action between a child and an adult or older person that results in some sort of sexual stimulation/gratification of the adult or older person at the expense of the child.

Neglect of Care: Neglect of care refers to the omission of normal expected care of the child. This includes neglecting the child by not making sure she has food, clothing, health, education, proper supervision, and of course, love and attention.

What causes people to abuse or neglect a child?

Unfortunately, there is no simple answer. Factors that appear in situations of abuse may include poor impulse control (striking out in anger before thinking about it), financial stresses, job difficulty, or poor social interaction within the family. There is also some indication that a family history of abuse, mental illness, and poverty may be included in the causes of abuse. Parents with low self-esteem and who fear rejection may also be at risk for child abuse.

What sort of injury or trauma can result from child abuse?

A child or infant who has been physically abused can sustain any number of injuries ranging from a slight cut to permanent brain damage. The neglected and/or verbally abused child may be filthy, malnourished and sickly, or withdrawn—unable to socialize for fear of more abuse. Abuse may take almost any form— none of which is to be tolerated!

What is shaken infant syndrome?

Shaken baby or whiplash is a syndrome occurring when a child under one year of age sustains skull and long bone injury. When these children are first presented to the physicians, the actual injury may not be detectable, but rather misdiagnosed as meningitis or some type of seizure disorder. The injuries, however, have occurred by someone holding the baby by the chest and shaking vigorously. This can cause fractures in the extremities and will tear some of the vessels in the head, causing bleeding and swelling in the brain. Occasionally, some of these children will show an overt fracture, one that is readily discovered through examination because the baby's head was struck against a hard object while being shaken.

When these children are brought in by their parents, they may be having seizures or respiratory difficulty—this because the baby's lungs may have collapsed from the abuse. Some of the babies will show signs of hydrocephalus—enlarged head—due to slow-developing bleeding under the skull. Many times, parents have no obvious history of trauma and will insist that the baby has just had a fall; however, on further questioning, it is often revealed that there had been, in fact, past trauma or instances of abuse in their family history.

I have heard of Munchausen syndrome by proxy. What is this?

This is a relatively rare disorder that can best be described as a situation where a parent or adult actually *causes* their child to become ill, falsifying symptoms necessitating medical attention for the child. Because the histories are vague and difficult to document, it is extremely hard to identify this syndrome. Patients are taken from doctor to doctor in search of positive findings. In other words, these children are taken to doctors until one of them agrees with the parents that the child is actually ill! Some parents or caregivers have even substituted their own blood for that of the child in hopes of finding something abnormal!

Many times, if the child is actually admitted to the hospital, he or she will get better, but suddenly worsen again when discharge is near, or when back at home under the care of the abusing parent.

As you can see, this syndrome is very difficult to diagnose and must be approached with care and diligence by medical personnel.

What can I do to prevent abuse and neglect?

Obviously, there is no excuse for any type of abuse, regardless of the circumstances. After all, what could a child possibly do, *realistically*, to warrant being so disrespected? A child should not have to fear the people he loves!

In extreme cases of abuse—indeed ANY case of abuse—both the parent and the child must have immediate medical and/or psychiatric treatment. PERIOD. The child should be removed from the home, AT LEAST TEMPORARILY, and placed in a safe, comfortable environment. There should be no second chance for abuse!

Parents have to be aware of a potential problem developing in the home. If you feel that you might harm your infant, or that you may be neglecting you infant, see your pediatrician or your personal doctor. SEEK HELP! There are qualified professionals who can help you.

Prevention of abuse requires learning to alter your own behavior and should be done with qualified counselors who will not only work with the parents, but ultimately with the whole family.

Children deserve a fighting chance at life. They shouldn't have to fight for a chance! We, ALL of us, must take responsibility for this terrible situation, and stop hurting our children. It may take months or years in therapy, but you and your infant will be the beneficiaries.

Epilogue

Congratulations! You've done it! You've actually made it through one of the toughest, most confusing, exasperating, yet wonderful years of your life, and you've started a brand new human being on the road to adulthood! By the end of the first year of life, you will likely have a difficult time recognizing the tiny infant you brought home from the hospital! The little scrunched up, totally dependent, mostly sleeping bundle you first held in your arms will have developed, seemingly overnight, into a real person!

How do you feel? I'm betting that even after all the diapers and bottles, fevers and coughs, earaches and colic, the things you remember *most* vividly are the smiles and chuckles, squeals and laughter, baby smells and soft skin, and those never-to-be-forgotten expressions traveling across your baby's face as he (or she) learns that having *you* as a parent is a pretty great thing!

Some of the most important lessons you've learned during this first year probably have to do less with the physical, hands-on aspect of caring for your child (those things come naturally with practice) than with the satisfaction you should feel knowing that your persistence, patience, and willingness to learn has allowed you to accomplish something you can be very proud of—getting through this first year with your new baby! (And if your baby has not yet been born, I sincerely hope this book has given you some practical, simple advice that will serve you well as you prepare for the wonder of parenthood!)

Remember that babies are complicated miracles.

Appendix

References

Adoption

* Brodzinsky, A. 1986. *The Mulberry Bird: Story of Adoption.* Fort Wayne, Ind.: Perspective Press.

* Freudberg, J., and T. Geiss. 1986. *Susan and Gordon Adopt a Baby.* New York: Random House/Children's Television Workshop.

Breast-feeding

American Academy of Pediatrics Committee on Drugs. 1994. *Pediatrics* 93:137.

Barnes, G. R., A. N. Lethin, E. B. Jackson, et al. 1953. Management of breast feeding. *Journal of the American Medical Association* 151:192.

* Eiger, M. S., and S. W. Olds. 1987. *The Complete Book of Breastfeeding.* New York: Workman Publishing.

Gray-Donald. K., M. S. Kramer, S. Munday, et al. 1985. Effect of formula supplementation in the hospital on the duration of breast feeding: A controlled clinical trial. *Pediatrics* 75:514.

Herrara, A. J. 1984. Supplemental versus unsupplemented breast-feeding. *Perinatology Neonatology* 8:70.

---

* Indicates parent reading material.

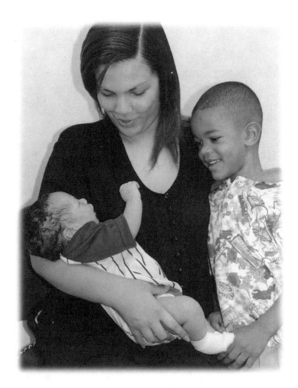

Lawrence, R. A. 1994. *Breastfeeding: A Guide for the Medical Profession*, 4th ed. St. Louis: Mosby-Yearbook Inc.

Piftenger, J. E., and J. G. Pittenger. 1977. The perinatal period: Breeding ground for marital and parental maladjustment. *Keeping Abreast Journal* 2:18.

* Rosenthal, M. S. 1996. *The Breastfeeding Source Book*. Los Angeles: Lowell House.

Ryan, A. S., D. Rush, F. W. Krieger, and G. E. Lewandoski. 1991. Recent declines in breast feeding in the United States, 1984-1989. *Pediatrics* 88:719–727.

Stiehm, E. R., and P. Vink. 1991. Transmission of human immunodeficiency virus infection by breastfeeding. *Journal of Pediatrics* 118:410-412.

Subcommittee on Nutrition During Lactation. Food and Nutrition Board, Institute of Medicine. 1991. Washington, D.C.: National Academy Press

* Tamaro, J. 1996. *Breastfeeding Basics—So That's What They're For!* Holbrook, Mass.: Adams Media Corp.

Waletzky, L. R. 1979. Husbands' problems with breastfeeding. *American Journal of Orthopsychiatry* 49:349.

Child Abuse

Caffey, J. 1974. The whiplash shaken infant syndrome: Manual shaking by the extremities with whiplash induced intracranial and intraocular bleeding, linked with residual permanent brain damage and mental retardation. *Pediatrics* 54:396.

Dine, M. S., and M. E. McGovern. 1982. Intentional poisoning of children—an overlooked category of child abuse: report of seven cases and review of the literature. *Pediatrics* 70:32.

Dubowitz, H. 1990. Pediatrician's role in preventing child maltreatment. *Pediatric Clinics of North America* 37:989.

Panel on Research on Child Abuse and Neglect. 1993. *Understanding Child Abuse and Neglect.* Washington, D.C.: National Academy Press.

Wissow, L. S. 1990. *Child Advocacy for the Clinician: An Approach to Child Abuse and Neglect.* Baltimore: Williams and Wilkins.

Colic

Brazelton, T. B. 1962. Crying in infancy. *Pediatrics* 29:5795.

Carey, W. B. 1984. Colic: Primary excessive crying as an infant-environment interaction. *Pediatric Clinics of North America* 31:933.

* Waldman W. 1982. *Coping with Infant Colic: A Guide for Parents.* Columbus, Ohio: Ross Laboratories.

Cystic Fibrosis

FitzSimmons, S. C. 1993. The changing epidemiology of cystic fibrosis. *Journal of Pediatrics* 1221:1.

Kerem, E., et al. 1992. Prediction of mortality in patients with cystic fibrosis. *New England Journal of Medicine* 326:1187.

Delivery

American Academy of Pediatrics/American College of Obstetricians and Gynecologists. 1992. *Guidelines for Perinatal Care*, 3rd ed.

Apgar, V. 1953. A proposal for a new method of evaluation of the newborn infant. *Anesthesia and Analgesia* 32:260.

General Health and Development

Anders, T. F., et al. 1995. Normal sleep in neonates and children. In R. Ferber and M. Krygen, editors: *Principles and Practices of Sleep Medicine.* Philadelphia: WB Saunders.

---

* Indicates parent reading material.

Baraff, L. J., et al. 1993. Practical guideline for the management of infants and children, 0 to 36 months of age with fever without source. *Pediatrics* 92:1.

Coons, S., and C. Guillemault. 1984. Development of consolidated sleep and wakeful periods in relation to the day/night cycle of infancy. *Developmental Medicine and Child Neurology* 26:169–176.

Fox, J. A., et al. 1997. *Primary Health Care of Children.* St. Louis: Mosby-Yearbook Inc,

Hamill, P. V. V., T. A. Drizd, et al. 1979. Physical growth: National Center for Health Statistics Percentiles. *American Journal of Clinical Nutrition* 32:607–629.

Hoekelman, R. A., et al. 1997. *Primary Pediatric Care,* 3rd ed. St. Louis: Mosby-Yearbook Inc.

Lowrey, G. H. 1986. *Growth and Development of Children,* 8th ed. St. Louis: Mosby-Yearbook Inc.

Oski, F., et al. 1994. *Principles and Practice of Pediatrics.* 2nd ed. 1994. Philadelphia: JB Lippincott Co.

Santrock, J. 1995. *Life-Span Development,* 5th ed. Dubuque, Iowa: Wm C. Brown Communications Inc.

Weston, R. L., et al. 1996. *Color Textbook of Pediatric Dermatology,* 2nd ed. St. Louis: Mosby-Yearbook Inc.

HIV

American Academy of Pediatrics Provisional Committee on Pediatric AIDS. 1995. Perinatal human immunodeficiency virus testing. *Pediatrics* 95:303–307.

Immunizations

Advisory Committee on Immunization Practices (ACIP), U.S. Public Health Service. 1995. Recommendations published annually in *Morbidity and Mortality Weekly Report* (MMWR). 43:959–960

American Academy of Pediatrics, Committee on Infectious Diseases. 1997. *Red book: Report of the Committee on Infectious Diseases,* 24th ed. Elk Grove Village, Ill.: American Academy of Pediatrics.

American Academy of Pediatrics, Committee on Infectious Diseases. 1996. *Pediatrics* 97:143.

Lead Poisoning

U.S. Dept of Health and Human Services. 1991. Centers for Disease Control and Prevention: Strategic plan for the elimination of childhood lead poisoning. Atlanta, Ga.: U.S. Dept of Health and Human Services.

U.S. Dept of Health and Human Services. 1991. Public Health Service, Centers for Disease Control and Prevention: Preventing lead poisoning in young children. Atlanta, Ga.: U.S. Dept of Health and Human Services.

Miscellaneous

American Academy of Pediatrics, Committee on Fetus and Newborn. 1985. Home phototherapy. *Pediatrics* 76:136.

American Academy of Pediatrics, Subcommittee on Hyperbilirubinemia. 1994. Management of hyperbilirubinemia in the healthy term newborn. Elk Grove Village, Ill.: American Academy of Pediatrics.

Anderson, G. C. 1986. Pacifiers: the positive side. *Maternal Child Nursing* 11:122.

Berg, R. W., K. W. Buckingham, and R. L. Stewart. 1986. Etiologic factors in diaper dermatitis: The role of urine. *Pediatric Dermatology* 3:102.

Buckingham, K. W., and R. W. Berg. 1986. Etiologic factor in diaper dermatitis: The role of feces. *Pediatric Dermatology* 3:107.

Cordova, A. 1981. The Mongolian spot: A study of ethnic differences and a literature review. *Clinical Pediatrics* 20:714.

Evans, A. G. 1944. Comparitive incidence of umbilical hernias in colored and white infants. *Journal of the American Medical Association.* 33:158.

Gergen, P. V., D. I. Mulladly, and R. Evans. 1988. National survey of prevelance of asthma among children in U.S.: 1976-1980. *Pediatrics* 81:11.

Morley, C. J., et al. 1992. Axillary and rectal temperature measurements in infants. *Archive of the Disease of Children* 67:122.

National Heart, Lung and Blood Institute, National Asthma Education Program. 1991. *Guidelines for the Diagnosis and Management of Asthma,* NIH Consensus Report No. 91-3042. Bethesda, Md.: National Institutes of Health.

Ogren, J. M. 1990. The inaccuracy of axillary temperatures measured with an electronic thermometer. *American Journal of the Disease of Children* 144:110.

Walker, S. H. 1967. The natural history of umbilical hernia. *Clinical Pediatrics* 6:29.

Weston, W. L., A. T. Lane, and J. A. Weston. 1980. Diaper dermatitis: Current concepts. *Pediatrics* 66:532.

*Indicates parent reading material.

Nutrition

American Academy of Pediatrics Committee on Nutrition. 1980. On the feeding of supplemental foods to infants. *Pediatrics* 65:1178.

Barness, L. A., et al. 1993. *Pediatric Nutrition Handbook.* Elk Grove Village, Ill.: American Academy of Pediatrics.

* Castle, S. 1992. The complete new guide to preparing baby foods. New York: Bantam Books.

* Coyle, R. 1987. *Baby Let's Eat.* New York: Workman Publishing.

* Karmel, A. 1995. *Small Helpings.* Santa Rosa, Calif.: Cole Publishing Group.

* Robertson, L., C. Flinders, and B. Rupenthal. 1986. *The New Laurel's Kitchen: A Handbook for Vegetarian Cookery and Nutrition.* Berkeley, Calif.: Ten Speed Press.

* Yntema, S. K. 1980. *Vegetarian Baby: A Sensible Guide for Parents.* Ithaca, N.Y.: McBooks Press.

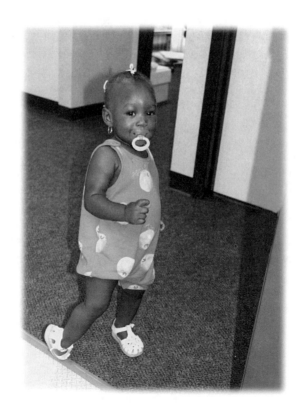

Parenting

American Academy of Pediatrics, Committee on Psychosocial Aspects of Child and Family Health. 1997. *Guidelines for Health Supervision*, 3rd ed. Elk Grove, Ill.: American Academy of Pediatrics.

* American Academy of Pediatrics. 1991. *Caring for Your Baby and Young Child: Birth to Age Five*. New York: Bantam Books.

* Brazelton, T. B. 1992. *Touchpoints: Your Child's Emotional and Behavioral Development*. New York: Addison-Wesley Publishing Co. Inc.

* Brazelton, T. B. 1972. *Infants and Mothers: Differences in Development*. New York: Dell Publishing.

* Chess, S., and A. Thomas. 1987. *Know Your Child: An Authoritative Guide for Today's Parents*. New York: Basic Books.

Klaus, M. H., and J. H. Kennell. 1983. *Bonding: The Beginnings of Parent-Infant Attachment*. St. Louis: Mosby-Yearbook.

Medoff-Cooper, B. 1995. Infant management: Implications for parenting from birth through one year. *Journal of Pediatric Nursing* 10:141–145.

Melvin, N. 1995. Children's temperament: Intervention for parents. *Journal of Pediatric Nursing* 10:152–159.

* Sears, W. 1991. *Keys to Becoming a Father*. New York: Barron's.

Premature and/or High-risk Infants

American Academy of Pediatrics. 1988. *American College of Obstetricians: Guidelines for Perinatal Care (Appendix B)*, 2nd ed. Elk Grove, Ill.: American Academy of Pediatrics.

Bronsteen, R., et al. 1989. Classification of twins and neonatal morbidity. *American Journal of Obstetrics and Gynecology* 74:98.

Kliegman, R., et al. 1996. The fetus and neonatal infant. *Nelson's Textbook of Pediatrics*, 15th ed., ed. R. E. Behrman, et al. Philadelphia: WB Saunders.

Papiernik, E., et al. 1985. Prevention of preterm babies: A perinatal study in Haguenau, France. *Pediatrics* 76:154.

Shiono, P. H., et al. Birth weight among women of different ethnic groups. *Journal of the American Medical Association* 255:48.

Shiono, P. H., et al. 1986. Ethnic differences in preterm and very preterm delivery. *American Journal of Public Health* 76:1317.

U.S. Dept of Health and Human Services. 1989. *Caring for Our Future: The Content of Prenatal Care*, Report of the Public Health Service Expert Panel on the Content of Prenatal Care. Washington, D.C.: U.S. Public Health Service.

---

* Indicates parent reading material.

Screening

Agency for Health Care Policy and Research, Sickle Cell Disease Guideline Panel. 1993. *Sickle Cell Disease: Screening, Diagnosis, Management and Counseling in Newborns and Infants.* Rockville, Md.: U.S. Dept of Health and Human Services.

Burton, B. 1987. Inborn errors of metabolism: The clinical diagnosis in early infancy. *Pediatrics* 79:359.

Committee on Genetics. 1994. Prenatal genetic diagnosis for pediatricians. *Pediatrics* 93:1010.

Committee on Genetics. 1992. Issues in newborn screening. *Pediatrics* 89:345.

Dworkin, P. H. 1989. British and American recommendations for developmental monitoring: The role of surveillance. *Pediatrics* 84:1000–1010.

Kennedy, C., et al. 1991. Otoacoustic emissions and auditory brainstem responses in the newborn. *Archive of the Disease of Children* 66:1124.

Northern, J. L., and D. Hayes. 1994. Universal screening for hearing impairment: Necessary, beneficial and justifiable. *Audiology Today* 6:10.

U.S. Preventive Services Task Force. 1996. *Guide to Clinical Preventive Services,* 2nd ed. Baltimore: Williams & Wilkins Co.

SIDS

American Academy of Pediatrics. 1992. Task force on infant positioning and SIDS. *Pediatrics.* 90:1120.

Kraus, J. F., S. Greenland, and M. Bulterys. 1989. Risk factors for SIDS in the U.S.: Collaborative Perinatal Project. *International Journal of Epidemiology* 18:113.

Substance Abuse

Azuma, S. D., et al. 1993. Outcome of children prenatally exposed to cocaine and other drugs: A path analysis of three year data. *Pediatrics* 92:396.

Committee on Substance Abuse, American Academy of Pediatrics. 1993. Role of the pediatrician in prevention and management of substance abuse. *Pediatrics.* 91:1010.

Day N. L., et al. 1993. The epidemiology of alcohol, marijuana, and cocaine use among women of childbearing age and pregnant women. *Clinincal Obstetrics and Gynecology* 36:232.

Hans, S. L. 1992. *Maternal Opioid Drug Use and Child Development in Maternal Substance Abuse and Developing Nervous System.* Chicago: Academic Press.

Jones, K. L., D. W. Smith, C. N. Ulleland, and A. P. Streissguth. 1973. Pattern of malformation in offspring of chronic alcoholic mothers. *Lancet* 1:1267–1271.

Naeye, R. L., et al. 1969. Fetal-complications of maternal heroin addiction, abnormal growth, infections and episodes of stress. *Journal of Pediatrics* 75:945.

Stone, M. L., et al. 1971. Narcotic addiction in pregnancy. *American Journal of Obstetrics and Gynecology* 109:716,1971.

Teeth

Chan, J. T., L. E. Wyborny, and D. S. 1990. Clinical applications of fluorides, *Clinical Dentistry*, ed. J. F. Hardin. Philadelphia: JB Lippincott.

Johnson, D. 1988. Baby bottle tooth decay: A preventable health problem in infants, *Update in Pediatric Dentistry*, 2nd ed. Pennsylvania: Professional Audience Communications, Inc.

Logan, W. G. H., and R. Krenfeld. 1933. Development of the human jaws and surrounding structures from birth to the age of fifteen years. *Journal of the American Dental Association* 20:379.

Von Burg, M., B. Sanders, and J. Weddell. 1995. Baby bottle tooth decay: A concern for all mothers. *Journal of Pediatric Nursing* 21(6):515–519.

Resources

Adoption

* National Council on Adoption
2025 M St. NW, Ste. 512
Washington, D.C. 20036
202-328-8072

Child Abuse and Neglect

* Child Help USA
(National Child Abuse Hotline)
800-422-4453

* National Committee for Prevention of Child Abuse
332 S Michigan Ave., Ste. 1600
Chicago, IL 60604
312-663-3520

---

* Indicates parent reading material.

Dentistry

* American Academy of Pediatric Dentistry
  211 East Chicago Ave.
  Chicago, IL 60611
  800-544-2174

* American Society of Dentistry for Children
  211 E Chicago Ave. Ste. 1430
  Chicago, IL 60611
  312-440-2500

Down's Syndrome

* National Down's Syndrome Society
  666 Broadway
  New York, NY 10112
  800-221-4602

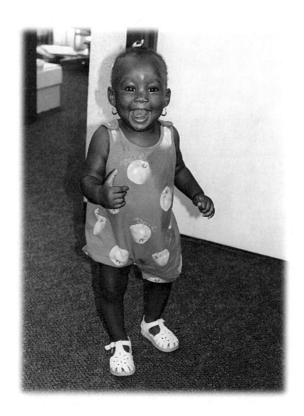

* Canadian Down's Syndrome Society
  501 18th Ave. SW #303
  Calgary, Alberta
  Canada T2T 0C7
  403-235-0746

* Asociación Méxicana de Sindrome de Down AC
  Boulevard de la Luz 232
  Jardínes del Pedrgal
  01900 México, DF
  525-652-4200

* Association for Retarded Citizens
  P.O. Box 6109
  Arlington, TX 76011
  817-261-6003

Parenting

* Active Parenting, Inc.
  810 Franklin Court, Ste. B
  Marietta, GA 30067
  800-825-0060

* Parents Without Partners
  401 N. Michigan Ave.
  Chicago, IL 60611-4267
  312-644-6610

Safety

Pamphlets may be ordered from:

* American Academy of Pediatrics Committee on Injury and
  Poison Prevention (1994): The Injury Prevention Program
  (TIPP)
  P.O. Box 927
  Elk Grove Village, IL 60009
  800-433-9016

* American Academy of Pediatrics
  Division of Publications
  141 Northwest Point Blvd.
  P.O. Box 927
  Elk Grove Village, IL 60009-0927
  800-443-9016

* Consumer Product Safety Commission
  Office of Information
  Washington, DC 20207
  800-638-2772

---

* Indicates parent reading material.

* Gerber Products Co.
  445 State St.
  Fremont, MI 49413
  800-595-0324

* Johnson & Johnson
  Skillman, NJ 08558-9418
  800-526-3967

* Mead Johnson & Co
  Evansville, IN 47721
  800-222-9123

* National Child Watch Campaign
  4065 Page Ave.
  P.O. Box 1368
  Jackson, MI 49204
  517-764-6070
  800-222-1464

* National SAFE KIDS Campaign
  111 Michigan Ave. NW
  Washington, DC 20010-2970
  202-662-0600

* Ross Laboratories
  Columbus, OH 43215-1724
  800-624-7677

Substance Abuse

* National Association for Perinatal Addiction Research and Education
  11 E Hubbard St., Ste. 200
  Chicago, IL 60611
  312-329-2512

* Center for Substance Abuse Prevention
  Rockwall Building 11, 9th Floor
  5600 Fishers Lane
  Rockville, MD 20857
  301-443-0365

Recommended Reading for Parents

General Baby Care

* Burck, F. W. 1991. *Babysense,* 2nd ed. New York: St. Martin's Press.
* Caplan, F., and T. Caplan. 1995. *The First Twelve Months of Life.* New York: Bantam Books.
* Leach, P. 1997. *Babyhood,* 2nd ed. New York: AA Knopf.

* Nathanson, L. W. 1994. *The Portable Pediatrician for Parents.* New York: Harper Collins Publishing.

* Neifert, M. 1986. *Dr. Mom.* New York: GP Putnam's Sons.

* Sears, W., and M. Sears. 1993. *The Baby Book.* New York: Little, Brown & Co.

* Shelov, S. P., et al. 1991. *Caring for Your Baby and Young Child.* New York: Bantam Books.

* Spock, B., and M. Rothenberg. 1992. *Dr. Spock's Baby and Child Care,* 6th ed. New York: Pocket Books.

* Indicates parent reading material.

Index

148; learning about parenting, 147-149; preparing babies for shots, 81; returning to work, 167-168; risk factors for SIDS and, 43; "rooming-in" after delivery, 25; self-doubt of, 148-149; self-identity and, 151-152; sex and new, 150-151, 156-157; sleep for, 40; sleeping with baby, 44; special care for by father, 160; teen parenting, 154-155. *See also* breast-feeding

mouth exam, 73

mumps, 80

Munchausen syndrome by proxy, 176-177

murmurs, heart, 76, 87

myelomeningocele, 84-85

N

neck exam, 74

neglect: resources for, 189; signs of in baby, 175-176

newborn rash (erythema toxicum), 138

newborns: assessments after delivery, 20-21; bonding with, 25-26, 155;checking baby's reflexes, 29-30; clothing for, 9; coming home from hospital, 33, 100-101, 148; delivery and, 19-20; effect of cocaine and heroin on, 173-174; eye and hair color of, 24-25; five senses at birth, 29; furniture for, 10-11; heart rate for, 76-77; with HIV, 93-94;holding, 31-32; ID band for, 20; medical concerns/problems for, 82-87; premature/low weight babies, 99; screening tests for, 22-23; SIDS and, 42-43; toiletries for, 9-10; Vitamin K for, 22; weight of, 19. *See also* development; holding babies

night-lights, 41

nose: cleaning, 36; clearing discharge from, 139-140

nurseries. *See* day care and nurseries

nutrition, 105-108; carbohydrates, 106-107; fats, 107; minerals, 107-108; proteins, 106; vitamins, 107. *See also* feeding

OPQ

obstetricians, 6-7

overfeeding, 111-112

pacifiers, 113

palmar reflex, 30

parenting, 147-177; with absent parent, 155; adoption, 164-165; baby's temperament, 161-162; bonding between father and child, 155; books about, 187; bringing your baby home, 148; by father, 159; changes for fathers, 155-156; child abuse, 174-177; coping with stress, 166-170; depression for fathers, 160-161; expressing anger, 170-172; fantasies and daydreams about baby, 148; fathers in delivery room, 158-159; fears and anxieties of new fathers, 157; house work by fathers, 157; learning about, 147-149; maintaining intimacy between partners, 156, 169-170; mother's role in family, 152; as partnership, 152; pregnancy and father's role, 158; quality time, 149; recommended reading about, 192-193; relational stress and, 160; resources on, 191; role models for children and, 162-164; role of father in family, 153; self-doubt and, 148-149; sex and, 150-151, 156-157; sharing chores, 167-168; special care for mother by father, 160; stress after baby's birth, 166-167; stress of single, 151-152, 153-154, 169; substance abuse, 172-174; for teens, 154-155

patent ductus arteriosus (PDA), 76

pediatricians: assessments of new-born after, 20-21; choosing, 7-8; exams of newborns, 24; mother's decision to breast-feed, 110; prenatal visits to, 12-15; questions for parent on first visit, 59; role of, 6-7; scheduling trips to, 33, 55-56; visits to, 58-60, 61, 62, 65, 67-87. *See also* physical examinations

penis: arranging during diapering, 37; circumcision of, 27-28; hy-pospadias, 86

perinatologist, 6

pertussis immunizations, 79

phenylketonuria (PKU), 23

physical abuse of child, 175

physical examinations: of chest, 74; of eyes, 72-73; of hands, legs, and feet, 77; of head, 69, 70-72; of heart, 76-77; immunizations, 78-82; of lungs, 74-75; monthly, 58-62, 65, 67-87; of mouth, 73; of neck, 74; questions to ask, 68; of sex organs, 77; of stom-ach, 75-76; weight and length of baby, 68-69

picking up baby. *See* holding babies

"pink eye," 93

pinworms, 95

plantar reflex, 30

plastic pants, 38

pneumonia, 89

polio immunizations, 80

pregnancy, father's role during, 158

premature apnea, 102

premature/low birth weight babies, 97-101; behavior of, 101; books about, 187; chances of, 97; com-pared with term infant, 99; eye care for, 99, 103; feeding, 100; holding and feeding, 100; hos-pital care for, 100; immuniza-tions for, 102; medical concerns/problems for, 101-103; reasons for, 98; special dif-ficulties for, 98-99; taking baby home, 100-101

prenatal visits to pediatrician, 12-15

projectile vomiting, 143

proteins, 106

pustular melanosis, 137

quality time with baby, 149

R

rashes, 137-138

reading to baby, 47, 66

rectal temperatures, 134-135

"red eye," 93

reflexes, checking, 29-30

REM (rapid eye movement) sleep, 44

resources, 189-192

respiratory distress syndrome, 102-103

retinopathy of prematurity (ROP), 103

ringworm, 95

risk factors: for premature/low weight babies, 98; for SIDS, 43

"rooming-in," 25

rooting reflex, 29

roseola, 96

rubella, 80-81

S

salmon patches, 137

salt, 108

scabies, 96

schedule for immunizations, 82

screening: books about, 188; for HIV, 94; tests for newborns, 22-23

seizures, febrile, 136

self-doubt of parents, 148-149

self-identity: new mothers and, 151-152; for single moms, 154

sepsis, 84

sex: interest of new mother in, 156-157; new father's view of part-

U

V

W

XYZ

Some Other New Harbinger Self-Help Titles